Bisphosphonates and Osteonecrosis of the Jaw: A Multidisciplinary Approach

Francesco Saverio De Ponte
Editor

Bisphosphonates and Osteonecrosis of the Jaw: A Multidisciplinary Approach

Foreword by Giorgio Iannetti

Springer

Editor
Francesco Saverio De Ponte
Unit of Maxillo-Facial Surgery
University of Messina
Messina
Italy

ISBN 978-88-470-2082-5 e-ISBN 978-88-470-2083-2
DOI 10.1007/978-88-470-2083-2
Springer Milan Heidelberg Dordrecht London New York

Library of Congress Control Number: 2011929633

Cover design: eStudio Calamar S.L.

Printed on acid-free paper

Springer is part of Springer Science+Business Media (www.springer.com)

With eternal gratitude to my teacher, to my parents for their tireless support, and to my children, who are my soul

Foreword

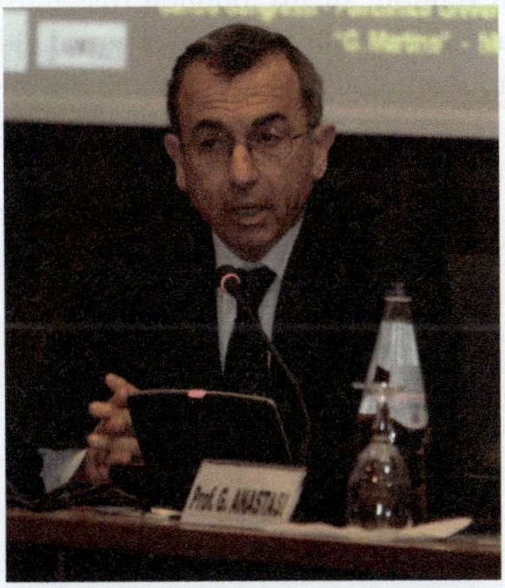

Prof. Giorgio Iannetti
Head of the Maxillofacial Surgery Department
University of Rome La Sapienza

The compilation of a volume on osteonecrosis due to bisphosphonates use (BIONJ) was motivated by the desire to translate into a single work the different experiences reported in the literature on this recent topic in research and clinical practice.

Prof. De Ponte must be credited for taking the initiative to create a text that was highly anticipated because of the importance and novelty of its subject matter. He also assumed responsibility for the organization of the chapters, which were written by colleagues who have dedicated themselves to this new and exciting multidisciplinary area of interest. Prof. De Ponte, with enthusiasm and expertise, has brought together their different points of views and research results to create a text that will guide and inform those who wish to engage in this specific field of medicine. From the first descriptions of the disease, by Marx in 2003, many aspects of BIONJ have been investigated, elucidated, and reported, but many others remain to be resolved. The definition, etiology, and clinical dynamics of BIONJ are complicated by the large and varied population of patients receiving bisphosphonates for the treatment of neoplastic and metabolic diseases. In addition, the different pharmacological effects of the numerous molecules belonging to the group called bisphosphonates add another variable.

These are the topics of discussion of the early chapters of the text, in which the pharmacological properties of bisphosphonates are defined and their use in three different populations, patients with cancer, patients with hematologic cancer, and those with osteo-metabolic disease, are described. The following chapters provide a comprehensive description of the clinical picture of BIONJ and a detailed overview of the diagnostic process and treatment of osteonecrosis. The final chapters address the prevention. In my opinion, the most effective preventative strategy for BIONJ, or any disease for that matter, is a multi-disciplinary approach, requiring close collaboration among all professionals working in this field.

In addition to sharing their experience and knowledge, the authors of *Bisphosphonates and Osteonecrosis of the Jaw: A Multidisciplinary Approach* highlight the many fascinating issues that remain to be explored regarding the study and treatment of BIONJ. This text will surely encourage the development of further knowledge and scientific research.

Rome, August 2011 Giorgio Iannetti

Contents

Contributors

Alessandro Agrillo Maxillofacial Surgery Department, University "La Sapienza" of Rome, Rome, Italy, e-mail: alessandro.agrillo@tiscali.it

Alessandro Allegra Division of Hematology, University of Messina, Messina, Italy, e-mail: alessandro.allegra@tin.it

Giuseppe Altavilla Medical Oncology Unit, Human Pathology Department, University of Messina, Messina, Italy, e-mail: galtavilla@unime.it

Giorgio Ascenti Department of Radiological Sciences, University of Messina, Policlinico "G. Martino", Messina, Italy, e-mail: gascenti@unime.it

Alfredo Blandino Department of Radiological Sciences, University of Messina, Policlinico "G. Martino", Messina, Italy, e-mail: ablandino@unime.it

Luigi Califano Stomatology and Maxillofacial Surgery, University of Naples "Federico II", Naples, Italy, e-mail: califano@unina.it

Luciano Catalfamo Unit of Maxillo-Facial Surgery, University of Messina, Messina, Italy, e-mail: lc.lab@libero.it

Annamaria Colao Endocrinology and Oncology Molecular and Clinical, University of Naples "Federico II", Naples, Italy, e-mail: calao@unina.it

Giuseppina Cutroneo Department of Biomorphology and Biotechnologies, University of Messina, c/o A.O.U. Policlinico Universitario "G. Martino", Messina, Italy, e-mail: gcutroneo@unime.it

Santino Ferrara Stomatology and Maxillofacial Surgery, University of Naples "Federico II", Naples, Italy, e-mail: ferraramaxillo@libero.it

Marco Friscia Department of Maxillo facial Surgery, University of Naples "Federico II", Naples, Italy, e-mail: marcofriscia@yahoo.it

Michele Gaeta Department of Radiological Sciences, University of Messina, Policlinico "G. Martino", Messina, Italy, e-mail: mgaeta@unime.it

Stefania Leuci Oral Medicine Unit, Department of Odontostomatological Sciences, University of Naples "Federico II", Naples, Italy, e-mail: stefania.leuci @unina.it

Giuseppe Lombardo Unit of Maxillofacial Surgery, G. Martino Polyclinic, University of Messina, Messina, Italy, e-mail: lombardo_peppe@libero.it

Grazia Marabello Medical Oncology Unit, Human Pathology Department, University of Messina, Messina, Italy, e-mail: gmarabello@unime.it

Claudio Marchetti Unit of Oral and Maxillofacial Surgery, Department of Oral Sciences, S. Orsola Hospital, University of Bologna, Bologna, Italy, e-mail: claudio.marchetti@unibo.it

Robert E. Marx Chief of the Division of Oral and Maxillofacial Surgery, University of Miami Miller School of Medicine, Miami, FL, USA, e-mail: rmarx@med.miami.edu

Silvio Mazziotti Department of Radiological Sciences, University of Messina, Policlinico "G. Martino", Messina, Italy, e-mail: smazziotti@unime.it

Achille Mileto Department of Radiological Sciences, University of Messina, Policlinico "G. Martino", Messina, Italy, e-mail: achille.mileto@gmail.com

Letteria Minutoli Department of Clinical and Experimental Medicine and Pharmacology, Section of Pharmacology, Faculty of Medicine and Surgery, Policlinico Universitario "G. Martino", Messina, Italy, e-mail: lminutoli@unime.it

Michele Davide Mignogna Oral Medicine Unit, Department of Odontostomatological Sciences, University of Naples "Federico II", Naples, Italy, e-mail: mignogna@unina.it

Filippo Moretti Unit of Oral and Maxillofacial Surgery, Department of Oral Sciences, S. Orsola Hospital, University of Bologna, Bologna, Italy, e-mail: filippo.moretti5@unibo.it

Caterina Musolino Division of Hematology, University of Messina, Messina, Italy, e-mail: cmusolino@unime.it

Carla Nava Unit of Maxillofacial Surgery, University of Messina, Messina, Italy, Unit of Maxillofacial Surgery, G. Martino Polyclinic, University of Messina, Messina, Italy, e-mail: carla.nava@libero.it

Giacomo Oteri Department of Dentistry, University of Messina, Messina, Italy, e-mail: giacomo.oteri@unime.it

Gian Andrea Pelliccioni Unit of Oral and Maxillofacial Surgery, Department of Oral Sciences, S. Orsola Hospital, University of Bologna, Bologna, Italy, e-mail: gian.pelliccioni@unibo.it

Vincenzo Pitini Medical Oncology Unit, Human Pathology Department, University of Messina, Messina, Italy, e-mail: vpitiui@unime.net

Salvatore L. Ruggiero New York Center for Orthognathic and Maxillofacial Surgery, Department of Oral and Maxillofacial Surgery, Stony Brook School of Dental Medicine, Lake Success, NY, USA, e-mail: sruggie@optonline.net

Francesco Saverio De Ponte Unit of Maxillofacial Surgery, G. Martino Polyclinic, University of Messina, Messina, Italy, e-mail: fdeponte@unime.it

Ignazio Salamone Department of Radiological Sciences, University of Messina, Policlinico "G. Martino", Messina, Italy

Angelina De Sarro Department of Clinical and Experimental Medicine and Pharmacology, Section of Pharmacology, Faculty of Medicine and Surgery, Policlinico Universitario "G. Martino", Messina, Italy, e-mail: desarro@unime.it

Chiara Tomasello Medical Oncology Unit, Human Pathology Department, University of Messina, Messina, Italy, e-mail: chiara.tomasello@alice.it

Paolo Vescovi Sezione di Odontostomatologia, Azienda Ospedaliero-Universitaria di Parma, Parma, Italy, e-mail: paolo.vescovi@unipr.it

Carmela Visalli Department of Radiological Sciences, University of Messina, Policlinico "G. Martino", Messina, Italy

Laura Vuolo Endocrinology and Oncology Molecular and Clinical, University of Naples "Federico II", Naples, Italy, e-mail: lauravuolo@tiscali.it

Introduction

1

Robert E. Marx

Abstract

Beginning with the first reports in 2001 and continuing to the present time, exposed bone in the jaws and, more recently, femoral fractures caused by the toxic effects of bisphosphonates on osteoclasts have become epidemic. In less than 10 years, more than 1,100 publications have been published on bisphosphonates-induced osteonecrosis of the jaw (BIONJ). 16 organizations have produced position papers, and tens of thousands of individuals have been afflicted by this serious drug-induced adverse side effect. The predictability of BIONJ occurring in humans has long been recognized, in the historical accounts of the phossy jaw epidemic between 1850 and 1906 and in the disease of osteopetrosis. BIONJ, as well as both of these pathologies, results from the over suppression of bone turnover (renewal), such that brittle and often necrotic bone develops in areas of the skeleton subject to the highest turnover in response to compressive forces and bending forces (e.g., alveolar bone in the jaws and the mid femur). The current challenge to clinicians is not to be ambivalent concerning the cause of BIONJ, as it is due to the bisphosphonate molecule itself, with all other medical conditions and drugs playing only contributing roles as co-morbidities. Accordingly, both the dose and the frequency of administration must be moderated. In addition, dental/oral and maxillofacial surgical teams must be able to competently manage and treat these individuals to control or resolve the disease.

R. E. Marx (✉)
Chief of the Division of Oral and Maxillofacial Surgery,
University of Miami Miller School of Medicine, Miami, FL, USA
e-mail: rmarx@med.miami.edu

F. S. De Ponte (ed.), *Bisphosphonates and Osteonecrosis of the Jaw: A Multidisciplinary Approach*, DOI: 10.1007/978-88-470-2083-2_1,

1.1 Introduction

Bisphosphonate-induced osteonecrosis of the jaws (BIONJ) in humans was first discussed in the textbook *Oral and Maxillofacial Pathology: A Rationale for the Diagnosis and Treatment* by Marx and Stern in 2001 [1]. At that time, this author incorrectly referred to this condition as an avascular necrosis because the exposed bone was indeed necrotic and did not bleed upon cutting into it (Fig. 1.1). In 2003, this author published the first journal report, entitled "Pamidronate (Aredia) and zolendronate (Zometa) induced avascular necrosis of the jaws: a growing epidemic" [2]. Labeling this clinical identity as "a growing epidemic" became a true prophecy, as Ruggerio et al. [3] soon thereafter published a 63 case experience and many other publications quickly followed [4–9]. Indeed, since 2003, there have been over 1,100 scientific publications about BIONJ, reporting over 12,000 cases with a nearly worldwide distribution. Over 16 dental and medical organizations have published position papers on this one topic [10, 11] and it has been the single most cited topic in the scientific literature since 2006.

Like other epidemics, such as the HIV epidemic of the 1980s and the phossy jaw epidemic between 1850 and 1906, there have been denials of the very existence of BIONJ by the respective drug companies, including denial of its importance and risks to patients. Another problem has been the inaccurate terminology used to describe BIONJ [10–13].

One should recall that the strange finding of immune shutdown and death by opportunistic infections in 1980, due to what we now know as HIV infection leading to AIDS, was initially denied and attributed to homosexual behavior and Haitian origins. In addition, HIV infection leading to AIDS was also given incorrect names, such as human T-cell lymphotropic virus I and II, neither of which actually causes AIDS, as well as names such as AIDS-related complex (ARC) [14]. Similarly, the original phossy jaw epidemic, most prominent in the UK and the USA, was also denied by the match-factory owners, who refused to recognize their role in a disease causing severe disabilities and a mortality of 20% (Fig. 1.2) [15].

1.2 The Phossy Jaw Epidemic of ~1850–1906

If BIONJ represents the second epidemic of phossy jaw, it is worthy reviewing the original epidemic. Although matches were invented in 1826, they were not widely used due to the poor lighting quality of the antimony sulfide and potassium chlorate in the match heads. However, in 1832, clever chemists added white phosphorous because it had a lower ignition temperature. These matches lit easily, even by abrading them on a pant leg or with the flick of a fingernail, and thus became enormously popular. By 1835, numerous match factories arose, producing what was called "strike anywhere matches" (Fig. 1.3). The match-factory workers, referred to as "mixers," worked 15-hour days over large heated vats of white

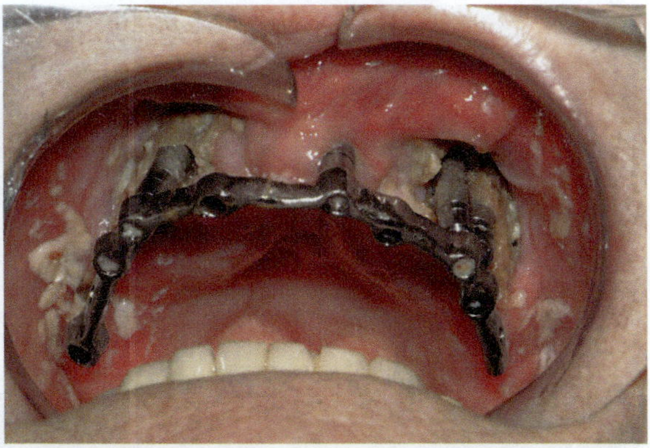

Fig. 1.1 One of the first cases of bisphosphonate-induced osteonecrosis of the jaws, with exposed necrotic bone that did not bleed

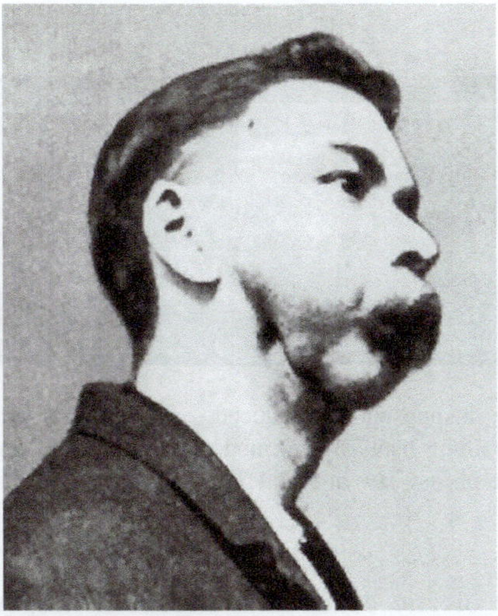

Fig. 1.2 Match-factory worker 1899. Phossy jaw causes fistulas and collapse of the mandible most likely due to a pathologic fracture

phosphorus, breathing in the vapors. Proportional to the length of time they worked in the match factory, many of the mixers developed exposed bone in the jaws that failed to heal, became secondarily infected, and produced draining fistulae just like those seen in many modern-day BIONJ patients (Fig. 1.4a, b) [15, 16]. A few of these workers also developed spontaneous leg fractures of the upper leg (femur), much in the same way that alendronate (Fosamax) has now been shown to produce spontaneous subtrochantaric femur fractures in those using the drug for more than 6 years (Fig. 1.5) [17–19]. The match-factory owners insisted that the numbers of cases was smaller than the actual number or they

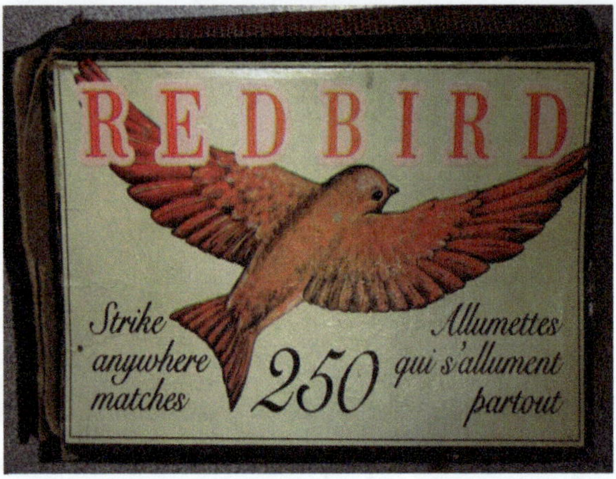

Fig. 1.3 "Strike anywhere matches" were popular because they would light easily due to white phosphorus in the match head

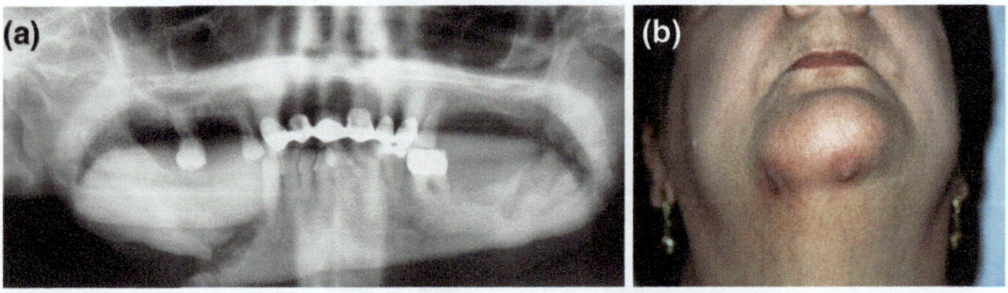

Fig. 1.4 **a** Modern-day bisphosphonate-induced osteonecrosis with exposed bone and a pathologic fracture. **b** Draining fistulas from modern-day bisphosphonate-induced osteonecrosis of the jaws similar to the phossy jaw in Fig. 1.2

denied the existence of any detrimental effects. In response, a strong popular movement arose to ban "strike anywhere matches" [20]. These cases and the public uproar concerning the deaths and disability caused by the matches led to the Berne Conference in Berne Switzerland and the banning of "strike anywhere matches" in 1906 [21].

Since then, rare cases of phossy jaw have been reported in fireworks- and munitions-plant workers whose jobs entail exposure to white phosphorus (P4O10). Additionally, phossy jaw and BIONJ have been linked by the demonstration that P4O10, when combined with water, carbon dioxide, and/or tetrahydrofolate in a one-carbon transfer, and with the amino acid hydroxylysine, all of which are common in the tracheo-bronchial tree, can produce a nitrogen-containing bisphosphonate eerily similar to pamidronate and alendronate, each of which has caused numerous cases of BIONJ (Fig. 1.6) [15].

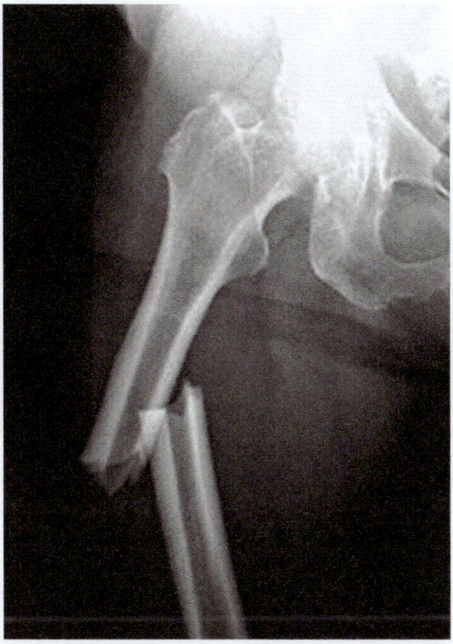

Fig. 1.5 Subtrochanteric femur fracture caused by alendronate (Fosamax) use over 7 years

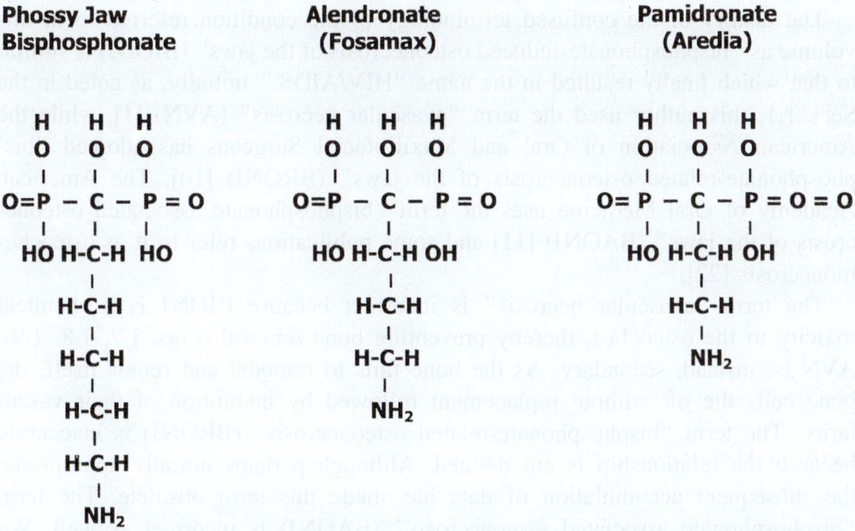

Fig. 1.6 Likely chemical formula of the phossy jaw bisphosphonate of the 1800s and the formulas of today's bisphosphonates pamidronate (Aredia) and alendronate (Fosamax)

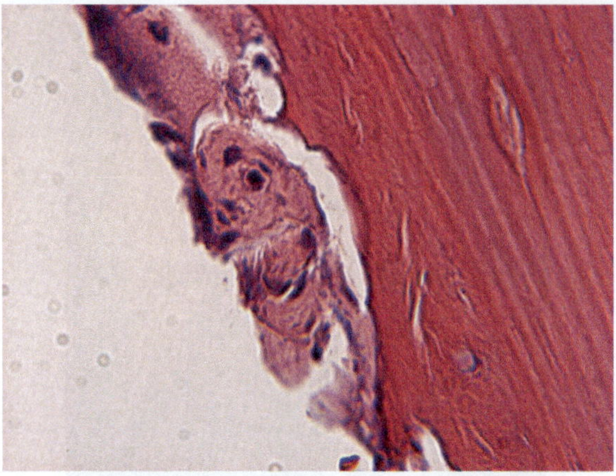

Fig. 1.7 Early toxic effects of bisphosphonate on an osteoclast. Note the cell's larger size, its numerous and disintegrating nuclei, and its separation from the sealing zone of Howship's lacunae

1.3 Correcting the Incorrect Terminology

As any new disease or drug complication becomes more fully recognized, the initial terms used in its description and typically adopted despite little scientific data or clinical experience, need to be revised.

The history of the confused terminology of the condition referred to in this volume as "bisphosphonate-induced osteonecrosis of the jaws" (BIONJ) is similar to that which finally resulted in the name "HIV/AIDS." Initially, as noted in the Sect. 1.1, this author used the term "avascular necrosis" (AVN) [1], while the American Association of Oral and Maxillofacial Surgeons has adopted "bisphosphonate-related osteonecrosis of the jaws" (BRONJ) [10]. The American Academy of Oral Medicine uses the term "bisphosphonate associated osteonecrosis of the jaws" (BAONJ) [11] and some publications refer to it as osteochemonecrosis [22].

The term "avascular necrosis" is incorrect because BIONJ is a chemical toxicity to the osteoclast, thereby preventing bone renewal (Figs. 1.7, 1.8, 1.9); AVN is, instead, secondary. As the bone fails to remodel and renew itself, the bone cells die off without replacement followed by involution of their vascularity. The term "bisphosphonate-related osteonecrosis" (BRONJ) is inaccurate because the relationship is not defined. Although perhaps initially appropriate, the subsequent accumulation of data has made this term obsolete. The term "bisphosphonate associated osteonecrosis" (BAONJ) is incorrect as well. We know that multiple odontogenic keratocysts are associated with basal cell nevus syndrome; however, the odontogenic keratocysts do not cause the syndrome but are a product of it. Analogously, while a low hemoglobin and low hematocrit may be related to anemia, they do not cause but are only signs of anemia, and

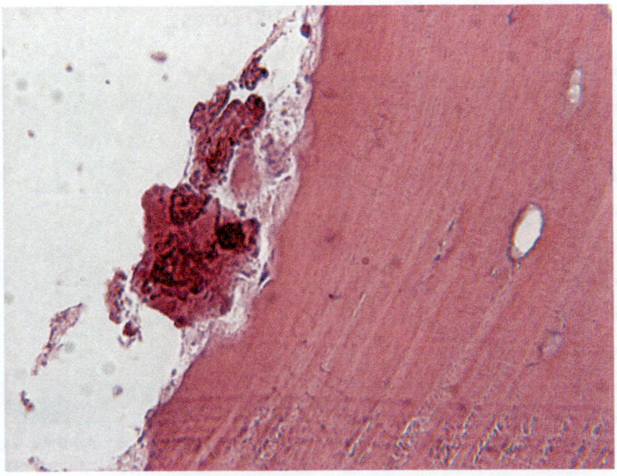

Fig. 1.8 Late toxic effects of bisphosphonates on osteoclasts. The dispersed chromatin and irregular cell membrane of an osteoclast in its last death throws are seen. The second osteoclast is only a contracted remnant of cytoplasm

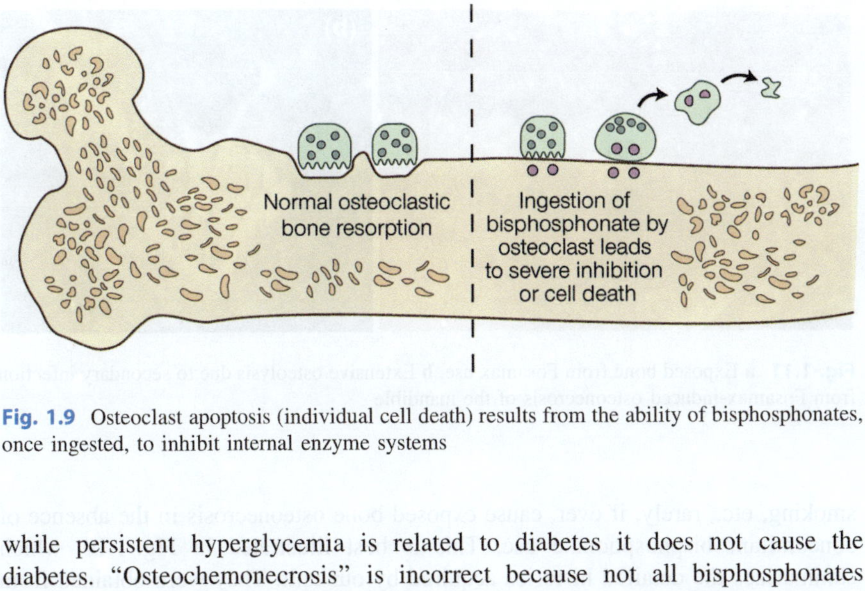

Fig. 1.9 Osteoclast apoptosis (individual cell death) results from the ability of bisphosphonates, once ingested, to inhibit internal enzyme systems

while persistent hyperglycemia is related to diabetes it does not cause the diabetes. "Osteochemonecrosis" is incorrect because not all bisphosphonates have activity against cancer cells. Even the claims that zolendronate has such activity have not been confirmed by independent studies and the drug is not approved as a direct chemotherapeutic agent nor does clinical experience support this off-label use.

No doubt "bisphosphonate-induced osteonecrosis of the jaws" (BIONJ) is the only correct term, as bisphosphonates are the proven causative agent. All the other reported risk factors, such as tooth extraction, tori, steroids, the cancer itself,

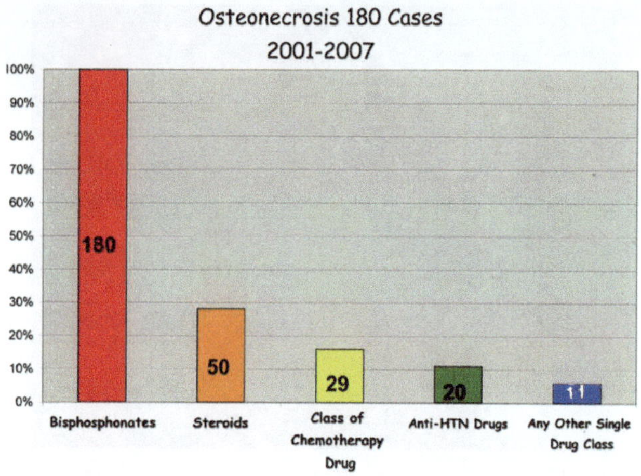

Fig. 1.10 Bar graph of 180 patients who presented with exposed bone in the mandible or maxilla related to drug exposures

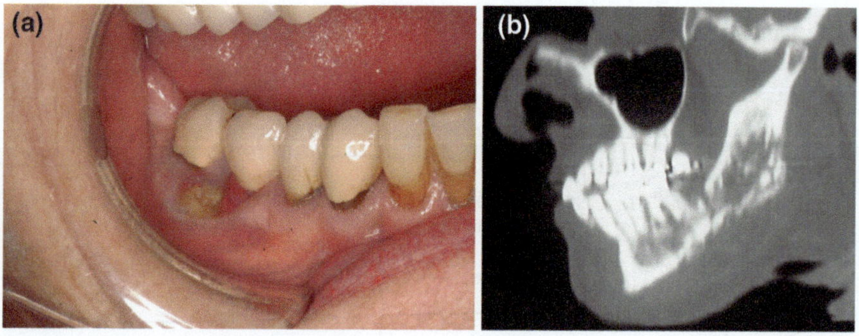

Fig. 1.11 **a** Exposed bone from Fosamax use. **b** Extensive osteolysis due to secondary infection from Fosamax-induced osteonecrosis of the mandible

smoking, etc., rarely, if ever, cause exposed bone osteonecrosis in the absence of concomitant bisphosphonate use. This is best illustrated in Fig. 1.10, which summarizes the detailed histories acquired by our unit. They were obtained from 180 consecutive patents reporting and confirmed upon examination to have 8 weeks or more of exposed bone in the mouth and no history of radiation therapy. All 180 patients (100%) had a history of bisphosphonate use or were actively taking a bisphosphonate. An examination of all other drugs and medical conditions found that the closest percentage of a comorbidity was 28% and involved steroids use (51/180; $p = 0.0001$).

1.4 Conclusions

The reality is that nitrogen-containing bisphosphonates are sufficiently potent to inhibit preosteoclast development in bone marrow and to kill mature osteoclasts when they begin to resorb bone [23]. They do this by irreversibly inhibiting the enzyme farnesyl synthetase, which is critical in the mevalonate pathway leading to geranylgeranyl proteins, resulting in osteoclast disruption in the presence of the high concentrations of bisphosphonate that may accumulate in bone [24]. As described elsewhere in this volume, bisphosphonates accumulate in bone by irreversibly binding to hydroxylapatite crystal and have a half-life in bone of over 11 years [25]. Their accumulation or more profound effect in the jaws is due to the fact that alveolar bone remodels at ten times the rate of the tibia and at five times the rate of basilar bone [26, 27]. This explains why BIONJ most always begins in the alveolar bone and may extend from there as a result of secondary infection. Likewise, BIONJ is more common in the molar areas, where greater stresses produce the need for alveolar bone remodeling (Fig. 1.11) [27].

The upcoming chapters will expound on this basic pharmacology and mechanism of action. The reader is advised to recall these basics, as they are the avenues used to establish prevention and treatment protocols as well as to understand the risk factors of each case.

As new bisphosphonates such as zolendronate, consumed once yearly for osteoporosis (Reclast) [28], come to the marketplace and other drugs appear with a similar mechanism of action, such as denosumab (Prolia), it is important to recall that any drug (bisphosphonates and denosumab) [29] or disease (osteopetrosis/marble bone disease; a genetic defect of osteoclast development) [30] that impairs normal osteoclastic function or reduces the osteoclast population will likely result in what has come to be recognized as "phossy jaw of the 21st century" [9].

References

1. Marx RE, Stern D (2002) Oral and maxillofacial pathology; a rational for diagnosis and treatment. Quintessence, Carol Stream
2. Marx RE (2003) Pamidronate (Aredia) and zoledronate (Zometa) induced avascular necrosis of the jaws: a growing epidemic. J Oral Surg 61:1567–1575
3. Ruggiero SL, Mehrota B, Rosenberg TJ et al (2004) Osteonecrosis of the jaws associated with the use of bisphosphonates: a review of 63 cases. J Oral Maxillofac Surg 62:527
4. Greenberg MS (2004) Intravenous bisphosphonates and osteonecrosis. Oral Surg Oral Med Oral Pathol Oral Radiol Endod 98:259–260
5. Migliorati CA, Schubert MM, Peterson DE, Seneda LM (2005) Bisphosphonate-associated osteonecrosis of mandibular and maxillary bone: an emerging oral complication of supportive cancer therapy. Cancer 104:83–93
6. Durie BGM, Katz M, McCoy L, Crowley J (2004) Osteonecrosis of the jaws in myeloma: time dependent correlation with Aredia and Zometa use. Blood 104(1):216a
7. Durie BGM, Katz M, Crowley J (2005) Osteonecrosis of the jaws and bisphosphonates. N Engl J Med 353:99–100

8. Bamias A, Kastritis E, Bamia C, Moulopoulos LA, Melakopoulos I, Bozas G, Koutsoukou V, Gika D, Anagnostopoulos A, Papadimitriou C, Terpos E, Dimopoulos MA (2005) Osteonecrosis of the jaw in cancer after treatment with bisphosphonates: incidence and risk factors. J Clin Oncol 23(34):8580–8587
9. Hellstein C, Marek C (2005) Bisphosphonate osteonecrosis (bis-phossy jaw): is this phossy jaw of the 21st century? J Oral Maxillofac Surg 63:682–689
10. Ruggiero SL, Dodson TB, Assael LA, Landesberg R, Marx RE, Mehrotra B (2009) American association of oral and maxillofacial surgeons position paper on bisphosphonate-related osteonecrosis of the jaws–2009 update. J Oral Maxillofac Surg 67(Suppl): 2–12
11. Migliorati CA, Casiglia J, Epstein J, Jaclosen PL, Sioegel MA, Woo SB (2005) Managing the care of patients with bisphonate associated ostenecrosis: an American academy of oral medicine position paper. J Am Dent Assoc 136:1658–1668
12. Tarassoff P, Csermak K (2003) Avascular necrosis of the jaws: risk factors in metastatic cancer patients. J Oral Maxillfoac Surg 61:1238–1239
13. Hoff AO, Toth BB, Altunday K, Johnson MM, Warnecke CL et al (2008) Frequency an drisk factors associated with osteonecrosis of the jaw in cancer patient treated with intravenous bisphosphonates. J Bone Miner Res 23:826–836
14. Kilby JM, Saag MS (1997) The pathogenesis of HIV-1 infection. In: Powserly WG (ed) Manual of HIV therapeutics. Lippincot-Raven, Philadelphia, pp 1–6
15. Marx RE (2008) Uncovering the cause of "phossy jaw" Circa 1858 to 1906: oral and maxillofacial surgery closed case files–cased closed. J Oral Maxillofac Surg 66(11):2356–2363
16. Simon J (1863) FIFO Report of the medical officer of the privy council. HMSU, London
17. Campston JE (2010) Bisphosphonates and atypical femoral fractures: a time for reflection. Maturitas 65:3–4
18. Shane E (2010) Evolving data about subtrochanteric fractures and bisphoshonates. N Engl J Med 362:1761–1771
19. Neviaser AS, Lane JM, Lenart BA, Edobor-Osula F, Lorich DG (2008) Low-energy femoral shaft fractures associated with alendronate use. J Orthop Trauma 22(5):346–350
20. Thorpe TE, Oliver T, Cunnigngham G (1899) Report on the use of phosphorus in manufacture of Lucifer mathches. HMSO, London
21. Miles AEW (1972) Phosphorus necrosis of the jaws: "phossy jaw". Br Dent J 133:203–206
22. Hellenstein JW, Marek CL (2006) Bisphosphonate induced osteochemonecrosis of the jaws. An ounce of prevention may be worth a pound of cure. Spec Care Dent 26:8–12
23. Van Beek ER, Lowe CWGM, Papapoulos SE (2002) Bisphosphonates suppress bone resorption by a direct effect on early osteoclast precursors without affecting the osteoclastogenic capacity of osteogenic cells: the role of protein geranlyations in the action of nitrogen-containing bisphosphonates on osteoclast precursors. Bone 30:64
24. Rogers MJ, Gordon S, Benford HL et al (2000) Cellular and molecular mechanisms of action of bisphosphonates. Skeletal complications of malignancy. Cancer 88(Suppl):2961
25. Lasseter KC, Porras AG, Denker A et al (2005) Pharmacokinetic considerations in determining the terminal elimination half lives of bisphosphonates. Clin Drug Invest 25(2):107–114
26. Dixon RB, Trickler ND, Garetto LP (1997) Bone turnover in elderly canine mandible and tibia. J Dent Res 76:2579
27. Vignery A, Baron R (1980) Dynamic histomorphometry of alveolar bone remodeling in the adult rat. Anta Res 196:191–198
28. Black DM, Delmas PD, Eastell R, Reid IR, Boonen S, Cauley JA, Cosman F, Lakatos P, Leung PC, Man Z, Mautalen C, Mesenbrink P, Hu H, Caminis J, Tong K, Rosario-Jansen T, Krasnow J, Hue TF, Sellmeyer D, Eriksen EF, Cummings SR (2007) Horizon Pivotal Fracture Trial. Once-yearly zoledronic acid for treatment of postmenopausal osteoporosis. N Engl J Med 356(18):1809–1822

29. Aghaloo TL, Feinsenfeld AL, Pretetradis S (2010) Osteonecrosis of the jaws in a patient on denosumab. J Oral Maxillofac Surg 68:959–963
30. Gorlin RJ, Cohen MM, Henneham RCM (2001) Syndromes of the head and neck, 4th edn. Oxford University Press, New York, pp 285–289

Pharmacology: Mechanism of Action of Bisphosphonates

2

Angelina De Sarro and Letteria Minutoli

Abstract

Bisphosphonates (BPs) are the most widely used and effective anti-resorptive agents for the treatment of diseases in which there is an increase in osteoclastic resorption, including post-menopausal osteoporosis, Paget's disease, and tumor-associated osteolysis. BPs are chemical analogs of inorganic pyrophosphate (PPi) and, although they share many pharmacological features with PPi, there are important biochemical differences, particularly in the way in which they bind to bone mineral and their effect on bone resorption. BPs are preferentially incorporated into sites of active bone remodeling, as commonly occurs in conditions characterized by accelerated skeletal turnover. These drugs can be grouped in three different classes: first-generation, non-nitrogen containing BPs (e.g., clodronate and etidronate), second-generation nitrogen-containing BPs (N-BPs, e.g., pamidronate and alendronate) and third-generation N-BPs (e.g., ibandronate and zoledronate) and the phosphonocarboxylate analogue 3-PEHPC. BPs have several common properties, including poor intestinal absorption, high affinity for bone mineral, inhibitory effects on osteoclastic bone resorption, prolonged bone retention, and elimination in the urine. They are generally well tolerated, even if side effects have been described.

A. De Sarro (✉)
Department of Clinical and Experimental Medicine and Pharmacology,
Section of Pharmacology, Faculty of Medicine and Surgery, Policlinico
Universitario "G. Martino", Messina, Italy
e-mail: desarro@unime.it

F. S. De Ponte (ed.), *Bisphosphonates and Osteonecrosis of the Jaw: A Multidisciplinary Approach*, DOI: 10.1007/978-88-470-2083-2_2,

2.1 Introduction

Bisphosphonates (BPs) are the most widely used and effective anti-resorptive agent for the treatment of diseases in which there is an increase in osteoclastic resorption, including post-menopausal osteoporosis, Paget's disease, and tumor-associated osteolysis.

2.2 Chemical Structure

Bisphosphonates are chemical analogs of inorganic pyrophosphate (PPi) and they are characterized by a phosphorus–carbon–phosphorus (P–C–P) backbone and two covalently bonded groups, R1 and R2, attached to the central carbon atom [1] (Fig. 2.1). The chemical stability of BPs and their resistance to enzymatic or acid hydrolysis is conferred by the carbon atom, which renders the molecule resistant to biological degradation and by the P–C–P structure, which imparts the ability to bind divalent metal ions, such as Ca^{2+} [2]. Moreover, R1 substituents, such as hydroxyl or amino, enhance chemisorption to bone mineral, while R2 substituents result in variations in the anti-resorptive potency of several orders of magnitude. The anti-resorptive potency observed with the different R2 groups is thought to be linked to their effects on biochemical activity, for example, inhibition of the enzyme farnesyl pyrophosphate synthase (FPPS), and to their ability to bind to hydroxyapatite [3].

2.3 Mechanism of Action and Pharmacodynamics

In humans, PPi is released as a by-product of many of the body's synthetic reactions; thus, it can be readily detected in many tissues, including blood and urine [4]. Pioneering studies from the 1960s demonstrated that PPi was capable of inhibiting calcification by binding to hydroxyapatite crystals, leading to the hypothesis that regulation of PPi levels is the mechanism by which bone mineralization is regulated [5]. Although the various bisphosphonates share many pharmacological features with PPi, important biochemical differences exist among them, particularly in the way in which they bind to bone mineral and their effect on bone resorption. Accordingly, bisphosphonate skeletal retention depends on the availability of hydroxyapatite binding sites. Bisphosphonates are preferentially incorporated into sites of active bone remodeling, as typically occurs in conditions characterized by accelerated skeletal turnover. They are rapidly cleared from the systemic circulation and deposited on bone mineral surfaces, particularly at sites of osteoclast activity. In fact, osteoclasts in the resorption phase are in a highly acidic microenvironment, which may facilitate bisphosphonate release from the bone surface, giving rise to high local bisphosphonate concentrations [2]. The bisphosphonate may then be internalized into the osteoclast, culminating in direct inhibition of osteoclast activity. This inhibition may be a consequence of a

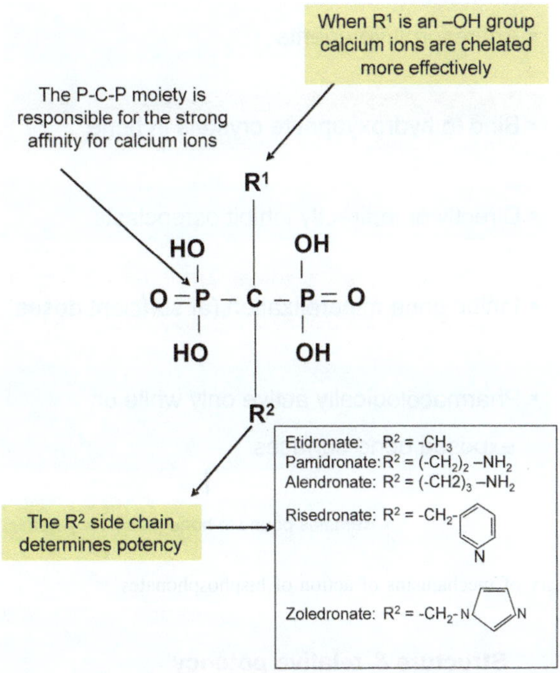

Fig. 2.1 Basic chemical structure of bisphosphonates

direct toxic effect involving osteoclast retraction, condensation, and cellular fragmentation, resulting in apoptosis. Alternatively, inhibition may be due to a disturbance of intracellular vesicular trafficking by the bisphosphonate [6], which may then lead, for example, to disorganization of the actin cytoskeleton and loss of actin rings or to disturbances of osteoclast ruffled-border formation [2] (Fig. 2.2).

Other cell types that internalize bisphosphonates by endocytosis are osteoblasts, macrophages, epithelial and endothelial cells, circulating monocytes, and neoplastic cells, such as myeloma and prostate tumor cells [7].

Based on recent discoveries concerning their molecular mechanism of action, bisphosphonates can be grouped in different classes: first-generation non-nitrogen-containing bisphosphonates (BPs), second- and third-generation nitrogen-containing bisphosphonates (N-BPs) (Fig. 2.3) and the phosphonocarboxylate analogue 3-PEHPC, previously known as NE10790 [8] (Fig. 2.4). First-generation BPs, such as clodronate and etidronate, are metabolized intracellularly to analogues of ATP. The intracellular accumulation of these metabolites within osteoclasts inhibits their function and induces apoptosis, very likely by inhibiting ATP-dependent enzymes [7]. In contrast, second-generation N-BPs, such as pamidronate and alendronate, and third-generation N-BPs, such as risendronate, ibandronate, and zoledronate, interfere with other metabolic reactions, notably those in the mevalonate biosynthetic pathway, by inhibiting farnesyl diphosphate (FPP) synthase. The inhibition of FPP synthase prevents the prenylation of small GTPases (e.g., Ras, Rho, Rab), which are

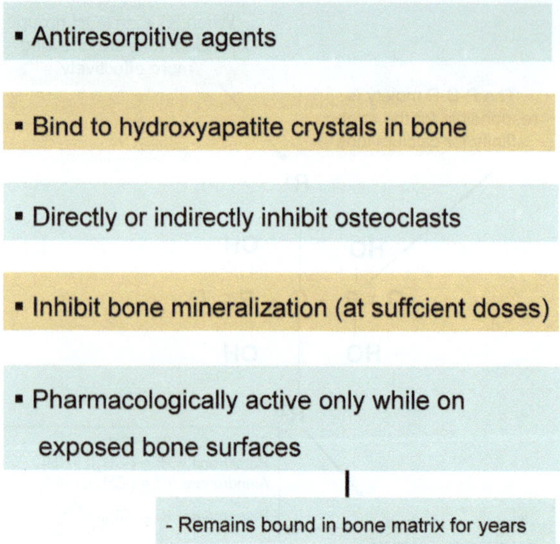

Fig. 2.2 Summary of mechanisms of action of bisphosphonates

Structure & relative potency of Bisphosphonates

Drug	R^1	R^2	Relative potency
Clodronate	Cl	Cl	1
Pamidronate (Aredia)	OH	$(CH_2)_2$–NH_2	10
Alendronate (Fosamax)	OH	$(CH_2)_3$–NH_2	100
Ibandronate	OH	$(CH_2)_2$–NCH_3 | $(CH_2)_4$–CH_3	500
Zoledronate	OH	CH_2–	1000

Fig. 2.3 Bisphosphonates are classified as first-, second-, and third-generation, implying progressively greater potencies. Clodronate is in the first category, pamidronate and alendronate in the second, and zoledronate in the third

important signaling proteins (Fig. 2.5). Phosphonocarboxylate analogue of the bisphosphonate risendronate, 3-PEHPC, in which one of the phosphonate groups is replaced with a carboxylate group, inhibits other enzymes of the mevalonate

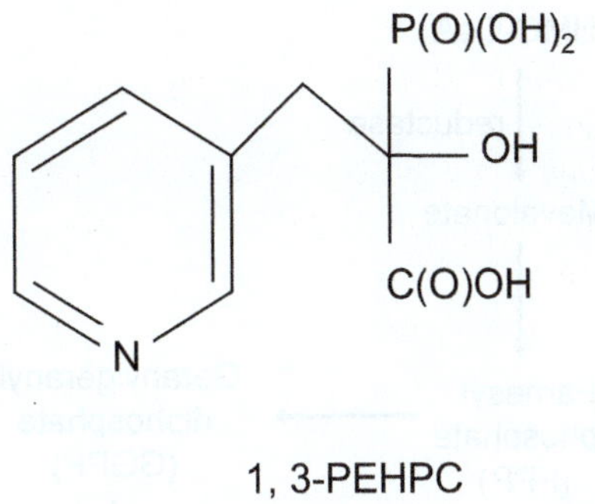

Fig. 2.4 Basic chemical structure of the phosphonocarboxylate analogue 1,3-PEHPC

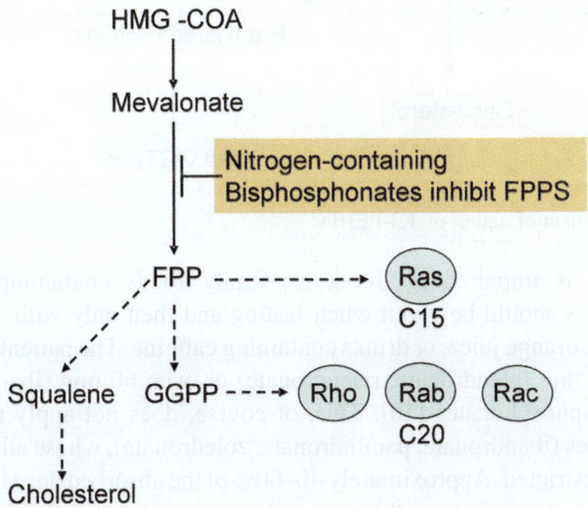

Fig. 2.5 Mechanism of action of nitrogen-containing bisphosphonates

pathway that use isoprenoid lipids (Fig. 2.6). In fact, 3-PEHPC specifically inhibits prenyl transferase Rab GGTase, thus preventing the prenylation and membrane localization of only the Rab GTPases, with no effect on FPP synthase. Due to the loss of one of the phosphonate groups, thus allowing the binding of only one calcium ion, 3-PEHPC is a comparatively weak inhibitor of bone resorption [8, 9].

2.4 Pharmacokinetics

Bisphosphonates have several common properties, including poor intestinal absorption, high affinity for bone mineral, inhibitory effects on osteoclastic bone resorption, prolonged bone retention, and elimination in the urine.

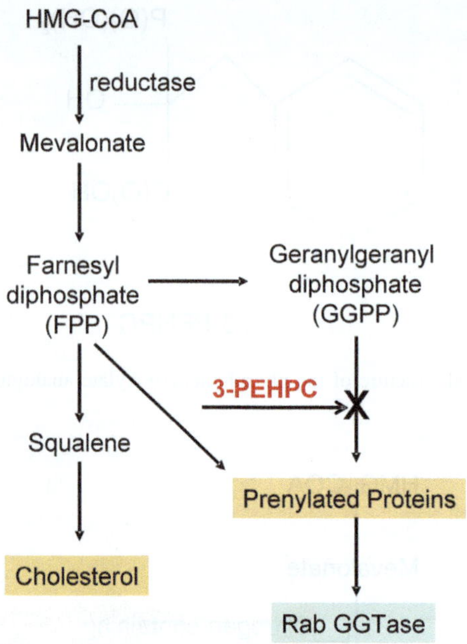

Fig. 2.6 Mechanism of action of 1,3-PEHPC

Absorption is impaired by food, especially foods containing calcium, so bisphosphonates should be given when fasting and then only with water, without dairy products, orange juice, or drinks containing caffeine. The patient should not eat for at least 30 min (alendronate, risendronate) or even 60 min (ibandronate) after taking oral bisphosphonates [10]. This, of course, does not apply to intravenous bisphosphonates (ibandronate, pamindronate, zoledronate), whose administration is not similarly restricted. Approximately 40–60% of the absorbed dose is concentrated in the skeleton, depending on the rate of bone turnover and the type of bisphosphonate, and the remaining amount is excreted, unaltered, in the urine [11]. The plasma half-life of bisphosphonates is short; given intravenously or orally, all bisphosphonates are eliminated quickly from the circulation, within 6 h of administration [12]. However, bisphosphonates stay embedded in bone for a very long time; for example, the terminal half-life of alendronate in humans has been estimated to be about 10 years [13]. Bisphosphonates may bind to plasma proteins, and some of them (especially N-BPs) are eliminated by a renal tubular secretory mechanism [11].

The suppressive effect of bisphosphonates on bone resorption is delayed by at least 1–2 days, in contrast to the more rapid effect of calcitonin. Both the concentration of bisphosphonate present in bone mineral at any time and the total dose administered over a long period of time seem to be important for the magnitude of the reduction in bone turnover [14, 15].

Drug interactions are limited to aminoglycoside antibiotics, in which case severe hypocalcemia can occur [16]. Calcium and magnesium salts impair the intestinal absorption of oral bisphosphonates.

2.5 Adverse Effects

Bisphosponates are generally well tolerated, but side effects have been described. Oral bisphosphonates (alendronate, risedronate, and ibandronate), mainly used for the treatment of osteoporosis, have been associated with adverse events involving the upper gastrointestinal (GI) tract, such as nausea, vomiting, epigastric pain, and dyspepsia, due to mucosal irritation of the upper GI tract. In fact, several cases of esophagitis with esophageal erosions or ulcerations associated with the use of alendronate were reported through post-marketing surveillance of the drug [17]. Accordingly, Barrett's esophagus should be a contraindication for bisphosphonates. Other adverse events are hypocalcaemia and secondary hyperparathyroidism, musculoskeletal pain, osteonecrosis of the jaw, atypical fractures of the femoral diaphysis, acute phase response (APR), and ocular events. The most common ocular side effect of bisposhonate is non-specific conjunctivitis [18], which usually improves without specific therapy and despite continuing treatment with bisphosphonates. However, the most serious ocular side effects are uveitis and scleritis, both of which require the discontinuation of bisphosphonate treatment [19].

Compounds in the group N-BPs are potent inhibitors of osteoclastic bone resorption. Six weeks after alendronate therapy is started, serum calcium and phosphorus decrease [20] and parathyroid hormone (PTH) significantly increases in a dose-dependent fashion. The increased PTH antagonizes the effect of bisphosphonates in bone and conserves calcium by increasing its tubular reabsorption in the kidneys and by stimulating the kidneys to produce 1,25-dihydroxyvitamin D.

Early clinical studies of bisphosphonates demonstrated strong anti-fracture efficacy for these agents. However, many investigators expressed concern that the anti-fracture benefit would be limited, because such striking reductions in bone remodeling might interfere with the microdamage repair process. This sequence of events did not seem to occur within the time frame of clinical anti-fracture trials, which lasted a minimum of 3 years and produced no evidence of resurgent fractures (femoral diaphysis) [21]. As reported by some authors, femoral-shaft fractures are rare among bisphosphonate users, suggesting that the osteoclasts of patients suffering from these fractures are genetically susceptible to over-suppression by bisphosphonates [22].

In 2008, an alert by the Food and Drug Administration (FDA) stated the following: "There is a possibility of severe and sometimes incapacitating bone, joint, and/or muscle (musculoskeletal) pain in patients taking bisphosphonates. The severe musculoskeletal pain may occur within days, months or years after starting bisphosphonates. Some patients have reported complete relief of symptoms after discontinuing the bisphosphonate, whereas others have reported slow or incomplete resolution" [23].

The transient flu-like symptoms produced by the APR sometimes occur after the administration of N-BPs and have been ascribed to the rapid and transient release of proinflammatory cytokines from circulating T cells [24]. APR is observed only rarely

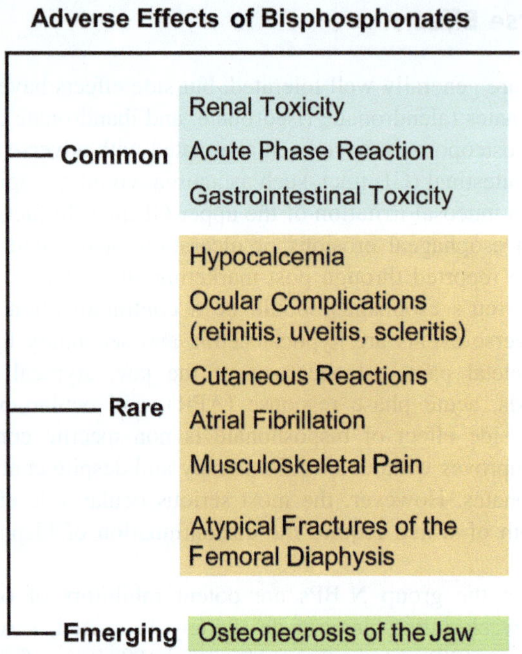

Fig. 2.7 Adverse events of bisphosphonates are classified as common, rare, and emerging

after intermittent oral therapy and more commonly following intravenous administration of bisphosphonates, including pamidronate, ibandronate, and zoledronate. The symptoms include low-grade fever, myalgia, headache, arthralgias, bone pain, and nausea; onset is usually within 3 days of drug administration, and symptoms generally resolve within 3 days of dosing but may last between 7 and 14 days. APR most often occurs in patients who have not previously been exposed to bisphosphonates and is unlikely to recur on subsequent dosing.

In 2002, the FDA received reports of several patients with cancer, treated with the intravenous bisphosphonate (zoledronate), who developed osteonecrosis of the jaw (ONJ) [25]. The risk of developing ONJ associated with oral bisphosphonates, while exceedingly small, appears to increase when the duration of therapy exceeds 3 years. This time-frame may be shortened in the presence of certain comorbidities, such as those associated with chronic corticosteroid use [26]. Potential preventive measures for bisphosphonate-related ONJ include: (a) a routine clinical dental examination before bisphosphonate therapy is initiated and, if possible, postponement of bisphosphonate therapy until dental treatment is completed; (b) discontinuation of oral bisphosphonates in asymptomatic patients, if systemic conditions permit, for a period of 3 months prior to and 3 months following elective invasive dental surgery; (c) specific treatments for patients with an established diagnosis of ONJ [27, 28].

Other side effects of bisphosphonates are cutaneous reactions [29], oral ulcerations, esophageal cancer [30], atrial fibrillation [31], and hepatitis [32]. Intravenous bisphosphonates (pamidronate, ibandronate and zoledronate), used in oncology and for the treatment of osteoporosis, have been associated with all of the above-mentioned adverse events, except those involving the upper GI tract. Moreover, pamidronate and zoledronate have been associated with renal toxicity [33, 34]. Generally, intravenous formulations are more potent than oral compounds and the frequency and severity of some of the bisphosphonate-associated adverse events are dose and potency dependent (Fig. 2.7).

Acknowledgment The authors thank Dr. Filippo Zagarella for his skilled technical assistance.

References

1. Rogers MJ, Gordon S, Benford HL et al (2000) Cellular and molecular mechanism of action of bisphoshonate. Cancer 88:2961–2978
2. Roger MJ (2003) New insights into the molecular mechanism of action of bisphosphonates. Curr Pharm Des 9:2643–2658
3. Russell RG (2007) Bisphosphonates: mode of action and pharmacology. Pediatrics 119: S150–S162
4. Russell RG (2006) Bisphosphonates: from bench to bedside. Ann NY Acad Sci 1068: 367–401
5. Chapurlat RD, Delmas PD (2006) Drug insight: bisphosphonates for postmenopausal osteoporosis. Nat Clin Pract Endocrinol Metab 2:211–219
6. Alakangas A, Selander K, Mulari M et al (2002) Alendronate disturbs vesicular trafficking in osteoclasts. Calcif Tissue Int 70:40–47
7. Roelofs AJ, Thompson K, Gordon S et al (2006) Molecular mechanisms of action of bisphosphonates: current status. Clin Cancer Res 12:6222s–6230s
8. Coxon FP, Ebetino FH, Mules EH et al (2005) Phosphonocarboxylate inhibitors of Rab geranylgeranyl transferase disrupt the prenylation and membrane localization of Rab proteins in osteoclasts in vitro and in vivo. Bone 37:349–358
9. Coxon FP, Helfrich MH, Larijani B et al (2001) Identification of a novel phosphonocarboxylate inhibitor of Rab geranylgeranyl transferase that specifically prevents Rab prenylation in osteoclasts and macrophages. J Biol Chem 276:48213–48222
10. Papapoulos SE (2001) Bisphosphonates in the management of postmenopausal osteoporosis. In: Marcus R, Feldman D, Kelsey J (eds) Osteoporosis, 2nd edn. Academic, San Diego
11. Barrett J, Worth E, Bauss F et al (2004) Ibandronate: a clinical pharmacological and pharmacoknetic update. J Clin Pharmacol 44:951–965
12. Cremers SCLM, Pillai G, Papapoulos SE (2005) Pharmacokinetics-pharmacodynamics of bisphosphonates. Clin Pharmacokinet 44:551–570
13. Russel RGG (2007) Determinants of structure-function relationships among bisphosphonates. Bone 40:S21–S25
14. Riis BJ, Ise J, von Stein T et al (2001) Ibandronate: a comparison of oral daily dosing versus intermittent dosing in postmenopausal osteoporosis. J Bone Miner Res 16:1871–1878
15. Tankó LB, Mouritzen U, Lehmann HJ et al (2003) Oral ibandronate: changes in markers of bone turnover during adequately dosed continuous and weekly therapy and during different suboptimally dosed treatment regimens. Bone 32:687–693
16. Liamis G, Milionis HJ, Elisaf M (2009) A review of drug-induced hypocalcemia. Bone Miner Metab 27:635–642

17. Levine MA, Grootendorst P (2000) Proportion of osteoporotic post-menopausal women at increased risk for upper GI adverse events associated with bisphosphonate therapy. Pharmacoepidemiol Drug Saf 9:367–370
18. Fraunfelder FW, Fraunfelder FT, Jensvold B (2003) Scleritis and other ocular side effects associated with pamidronate disodium. Am J Ophthalmol 135:219–222
19. French DD, Margo CE (2008) Postmarketing surveillance of uveitis and scleritis with bisphosphonates among a national veteran cohort. Retina 28:889–893
20. Maalouf NM, Heller HJ, Odvina CV et al (2006) Bisphosphonate-induced hypocalcemia: report of 3 cases and review of literature. Endocr Pract 12:48–53
21. Odvina CV, Zerwekh JE, Rao ES et al (2005) Severely suppressed bone turnover: a potential complication of alendronate therapy. J Clin Endocrinol Metab 90:1294–1301
22. Visekruna M, Wilson D, McKienan FE (2008) Severely suppressed bone turnover and atypical skeletal fragility. J Clin Endocrinol Metab 93:2948–2952
23. US Food and Drug Administration (2008) Information for healthcare professionals: bisphosphonates (marketed as Actonel, Actonel Ca, Aredia, Boniva, Didronel, Fosamax, Fosamax D, Reclast, Skelid, and Zometa), January 7, 2008. http://www.fda.gov/CDER/drug/InfoSheets/HCP/bisphosphonatesHCP.htm. Accessed 6 June 2008
24. Hewitt RE, Lissina A, Green AE et al (2005) The bisphosphonate acute phase response: rapid and copious production of proinflammatory cytokines by peripheral blood gd T cells in response to aminobisphosphonates is inhibited by statins. Clin Exp Immunol 139:101–111
25. Edwards BJ, Gounder M, McKoy JM et al (2008) Pharmacovigilance and reporting oversight in US FDA fast-track process: bisphosphonates and osteonecrosis of the jaw. Lancet Oncol 9:1166–1172
26. King AE, Umland EM (2008) Osteonecrosis of the jaw in patients receiving intravenous or oral bisphosphonates. Pharmacotherapy 28:667–677
27. Ruggiero S, Gralow J, Marx RE (2006) Practical guidelines for the prevention, diagnosis, and treatment of osteonecrosis of the jaw in patients with cancer. J Oncol Pract 2:7–14
28. Marx RE, Cillo JE Jr, Ulloa JJ (2007) Oral bisphosphonate-induced osteonecrosis: risk factors, prediction of risk using serum CTX testing, prevention, and treatment. J Oral Maxillofac Surg 65:2397–2410
29. Kontoleon P, Ilias I, Stavropoulos PG et al (2000) Urticaria after administration of alendronate. Acta Derm Venereol 80:398
30. Wysowski DK (2009) Reports of esophageal cancer with oral bisphosphonate use. N Engl J Med 360:89–90
31. Cummings SR, Schwartz AV (2007) Alendronate and atrial fibrillation. N Engl J Med 356:1895–1896
32. Halabe A, Lifschitz BM, Azuri J (2000) Liver damage due to alendronate. N Engl J Med 343:365–366
33. Ten Dam MA, Hilbrands LB, Wetzels JF (2010) Nephrotic syndrome induced by pamidronate. Med Oncol Sep 24 (Epub ahead of print)
34. Weide R, Koppler H, Antras L et al (2010) Renal toxicity in patients with multiple myeloma receiving zoledronic acid vs. ibandronate: a retrospective medical records review. J Cancer Res Ther 6:31–35

Use of Bisphosphonates in Oncology

3

Giuseppe Altavilla, Grazia Marabello, Chiara Tomasello
and Vincenzo Pitini

Abstract
Bone is the third most common site involved by metastasis, behind lung and liver. Bone metastases occur in almost all tumors and may be classified as osteolytic, osteoblastic, or mixed, according to the primary mechanism of interference with normal bone remodeling. In many cases, both osteolytic and osteoblastic processes are affected. The main goals in the management of patients with bone metastases are to treat the underlying malignancy and to intervene such that skeletal complications are avoided. Therapeutic options include surgery, radiation, chemotherapy, hormonal and biologically targeted therapies, and bisphosphonates. To date, bisphosphonates are the primary treatment option for reducing, delaying, and preventing the skeletal complications associated with bone metastases, thus maintaining and restoring patients' mobility and function and reducing pain. The mechanism of bisphosphonates action and the use of these drugs in breast, prostate, lung, kidney, bladder, and thyroid cancers are described.

3.1 Introduction

The vast majority of deaths from cancer are due to metastatic disease. Metastasis can be defined as the development of secondary tumors at a distance from a primary site of cancer. Malignant primary tumors can often be surgically resected, but the cells that gain the ability to migrate throughout the body, seeding and

G. Altavilla (✉)
Human Pathology Department, Medical Oncology Unit,
University of Messina, Messina, Italy
e-mail: galtavilla@unime.it

F. S. De Ponte (ed.), *Bisphosphonates and Osteonecrosis of the Jaw: A Multidisciplinary Approach*, DOI: 10.1007/978-88-470-2083-2_3,

Table 3.1 Incidence of bone metastases according to primary malignancy

Primary malignancy	Rate (%)
Breast	47–85
Prostate	54–85
Lung	32–48
Kidney	33–40
Bladder	31–42
Thyroid	28–60
Rectum	8–13

proliferating in distant organs, are often those that cause the most harmful effects and, it seems, are the cells most difficult to target therapeutically.

Bone is the third most common site involved by metastasis, behind lung and liver [1]. While bone metastases occur in almost all tumors, the primary cancers most likely to metastasize to the skeleton are those arising in the breast and prostate. Approximately 70% of patients dying from these diseases have evidence of skeletal involvement at autopsy. Carcinomas of the thyroid, kidney, and bronchus also frequently cause bone metastases and have a post-mortem incidence of 30–40%. By contrast, tumors of the gastrointestinal tract do so rarely, affecting only 5% of patients dying from these malignancies. The incidence of metastatic bone disease in patients with solid tumors is summarized in Table 3.1.

In multiple myeloma, bone impairment is the most frequent clinical feature of the disease, with over 80 % of these patients presenting with pain [2].

More than 80% of bone metastases are located in the axial skeleton, with the vertebrae, ribs, and hips as the most frequently involved sites [1].

The balanced activity of osteoblasts and osteoclasts is the basis for physiologic bone remodeling. Activated osteoclasts are responsible for the resorption of bone, while osteoblasts form bone at the same site [3]. Bone metastases are classified as osteolytic, osteoblastic, or mixed, according to the primary mechanism of interference with normal bone remodeling. In many cases, both osteolytic and osteoblastic processes are involved. Thus, the classic view of bone metastases as either osteolytic or osteoblastic acknowledges the two extremes of a process wherein both biological situations coexist, with a clinical prevalence of the one over the other [3]. The pathogenesis of osteolytic damage is far from elucidated. Osteolysis is mediated by osteoclasts and does not result from the direct action of tumor cells on bone. Bone-derived transforming growth factor beta (TGF-β) and the tumor-derived parathyroid hormone-related protein (PTHrP) seem to be the major mediators involved in osteolytic metastases [3]. Osteoclasts are activated through the action of receptor activator of nuclear factor kb ligand (RANKL) on the RANK receptor, which is expressed on the cell membrane of osteoclast precursors. Osteolysis is suppressed by osteoprotegerin (OPG), which inhibits RANKL binding to the RANK receptor [4]. The ratio of

RANKL to OPG regulates osteoclast activity. Both RANKL and osteoprotegerin are potential targets for therapeutic interventions against the formation of bone metastases.

The improved survival of cancer patients that has been obtained over the past 30 years through improved diagnostic and therapeutic interventions may determine a higher risk to develop bone metastases during the natural history of their disease. Consequently, the long-term effects of treatment on the skeleton have become an important clinical problem and a specific rationale for the use of bone-targeted treatments.

The main goals in the management of patients with bone metastases are to treat the underlying malignancy and intervene to prevent skeletal complications. Options include surgery, radiation, chemotherapy, hormonal, and biologically targeted therapies, and bisphosphonates.

3.2 Bisphosphonates in Bone Metastasis

Following their administration, bisphosphonates bind hydroxyapatite crystals of the bone matrix, reaching very high local concentrations in the resorption lacunae, where they are internalized by the osteoclasts. This results in the disruption of a number of biochemical processes crucial to osteoclast function and ultimately leads to apoptotic cell death [5]. The molecular mechanism of action of bisphosphonates has been well elucidated: nitrogen-containing bisphosphonates inhibit enzymes of the mevalonate pathway that are responsible for the post-translational modification of a number of proteins, including small GTPases such as Ras and Rho. The inhibition of farnesyl diphosphate synthase blocks the prenylation of proteins, leading to a loss of downstream signaling essential for osteoclast functioning [6]. Non-nitrogen containing bisphosphonates, such as clodronate, have a different mode of action and induce osteoclast apoptosis through the generation of cytotoxic ATP analogues [7].

Recent studies also suggest that bisphosphonates have direct apoptotic effects on tumor cells and that this effect is enhanced by a combination with other anticancer agents [7].

Bone metastases often lead to skeletal complications, such as pain, pathological fractures requiring surgery and/or radiation to bone, spinal cord compression, or hypercalcemia of malignancy. Many of these complications are associated with life-altering morbidity and can negatively impact survival times. Pathological fractures are the most common skeletal events, reflecting the fragility of these patients' bones and the burden of bone pain. Many patients will have to receive radiation to bone in order to treat bone pain and to prevent complications. Moreover, skeletal events are associated with a loss of mobility and social functioning, a decrease in the quality of life, and a substantial increase in medical costs [8].

To date, bisphosphonates are the key treatment option for reducing, delaying, and preventing the skeletal complications associated with bone metastases, thus maintaining and restoring patient's mobility and function in addition to reducing pain [9]. Health economic studies on bisphosphonates indicate that they are an effective treatment considering drug costs, quality of life benefits (especially due to bone pain reduction), and incidence and costs of skeletal complications [10]. Nonetheless, the choice of bisphosphonates for a given clinical setting should be evidence based [8].

3.3 Breast Cancer

Factors that negatively affect normal bone homeostasis in patients with breast cancer may be related to either the cancer itself or its treatment.

In patients with early breast cancer treated in the adjuvant setting, treatments are the predominant cause of bone loss and increased fracture risk; these include use of ovarian ablation or endocrine therapy and chemotherapy. Endocrine therapies enhance bone loss rates either by lowering estrogen levels, as ovarian suppression and aromatase inhibitors do, or by interfering with estrogen signaling (e.g., tamoxifen in premenopausal women). Some chemotherapeutic agents may directly affect bone, resulting in a rapid decrease in bone mineral density; however, indirect effects of chemotherapy, such as induced ovarian dysfunction in premenopausal women leading to premature menopause, are more common.

Moreover, approximately 70% of patients with advanced breast disease develop bone metastases and are subject to some of the highest rates of skeletal morbidity and poor quality of life.

For all of the above reasons, the most significant trials examining the efficacy of bisphosphonates have been performed in breast cancer patients with bone metastases.

Paterson et al. [11] reported a randomized study of 173 patients with bone metastases from breast cancer treated with standard anti-cancer treatment(s) with or without clodronate, an oral bisphosphonate. In patients who received clodronate, there was an overall 28% reduction in skeletal morbidity. Indeed, the greatest benefit was registered for a significant reduction in the total number of hypercalcemic episodes, in the incidence of vertebral fractures, and in the rate of vertebral deformity.

Conte et al. reported the results of a multi-center study that randomized 295 patients with breast cancer and bone metastases to receive chemotherapy with or without intravenous pamidronate (45 mg) administered every 3 weeks. The median time to disease progression in bone was increased by 48% in patients who received pamidronate (249 vs. 168 days); marked pain relief was reported by 44% of pamidronate patients and by 30% of controls. The infusions were well tolerated, with no major toxicities reported [12].

Two larger double-blind, placebo-controlled trials of 90 mg pamidronate infusions administered every 3–4 weeks in addition to chemotherapy or endocrine therapy confirmed the efficacy of pamidronate for patients with breast cancer and lytic bone metastases.

Theriault et al. [13] randomized 372 women with breast cancer who had at least one lytic bone lesion and who were receiving hormonal therapy to receive 90 mg of pamidronate or placebo. The skeletal morbidity rate was significantly reduced in pamidronate-treated patients. The proportion of patients with skeletal complications was 56% in the pamidronate group and 67% in the placebo group. The time to the first skeletal complication was longer for patients receiving pamidronate than for those given placebo. Pamidronate was well tolerated.

In a second randomized trial, by Hortobagyi et al., 380 women with stage IV breast cancer receiving cytotoxic chemotherapy and with at least one lytic bone lesion were given either placebo or pamidronate (90 mg i.v.) The median time to the occurrence of the first skeletal complication was greater in the pamidronate group than in the placebo group (13.1 vs. 7.0 months), and the proportion of patients in whom any skeletal complication occurred was lower (43 vs. 56%). There was a significantly lower increase in both bone pain and deterioration of performance status in the pamidronate group than in the placebo group [14].

Zoledronic acid is a highly potent, new-generation bisphosphonate that has demonstrated greater potency than pamidronate in preclinical testing and can be safely administered via a 15 min infusion. In a placebo-controlled trial in Japan, Kohno et al. randomly assigned 228 women with bone metastases from breast cancer to treatment with zoledronic acid or placebo every 4 weeks. Zoledronic acid reduced the rate of skeletal-related events (SRE) by 39% compared with placebo. The percentage of patients with at least one SRE was significantly reduced by 20% in the zoledronic acid group (29.8 vs. 49.6% for placebo). Zoledronic acid was well tolerated, with a safety profile similar to placebo [15].

Zoledronic acid was compared with pamidronate in a randomized, non-inferiority double-blind, phase III trial. The 1648 patients with either Durie-Salmon stage III multiple myeloma or advanced breast cancer and at least one bone lesion were randomly assigned to treatment with either 4 or 8 mg of zoledronic acid, administered via a 15-min intravenous infusion or 90 mg of pamidronate administered via a 2 h intravenous infusion every 3–4 weeks for 12 months. The primary efficacy endpoint was the proportion of patients experiencing at least one SRE over 13 months. The results showed that the proportion of patients with at least one SRE was similar in all treatment groups. Median time to first SRE was approximately 1 year in each treatment group. The skeletal morbidity rate was slightly lower in patients treated with zoledronic acid than in those treated with pamidronate, and zoledronic acid (4 mg) significantly decreased the incidence of event rate following radiation therapy to bone, both overall and in breast cancer patients receiving hormonal therapy. Pain scores decreased in all treatment groups in the presence of stable or decreased analgesic use. Zoledronic acid (4 mg) and pamidronate were equally well tolerated. [16] After 25 months of follow-up, zoledronic acid had reduced both the overall proportion of patients with SREs and the skeletal morbidity rate similar to pamidronate. Compared with pamidronate, zoledronic acid (4 mg) reduced the overall risk of developing skeletal complications, including malignant hypercalcemia, by an additional 16%. In breast carcinoma patients, zoledronic acid

(4 mg) was significantly more effective than pamidronate, reducing the risk of SREs by 20% and by an additional 30% in patients receiving hormonal therapy [17].

Ibandronate is a new, potent amino-bisphosphonate available in oral and infusion formulations. In a phase III study, Body et al. compared the efficacy of ibandronate with that of placebo as intravenous therapy in metastatic bone disease due to breast cancer. The 466 patients were randomized to receive placebo (n = 158), or 2 mg (n = 154) or 6 mg (n = 154) of ibandronate every 3–4 weeks for up to 2 years. The primary efficacy parameter was the number of 12 week periods with new bone complications, expressed as the skeletal morbidity period rate (SMPR). Bone pain, analgesic use, and safety were evaluated monthly. The results showed that the SMPR was lower in both ibandronate groups than in the placebo group; the difference was statistically significant for the ibandronate 6 mg group ($p = 0.004$ vs. placebo). Consistent with the SMPR, ibandronate 6 mg significantly reduced the number of new bone events (by 38%) and increased time to first new bone event. Patients on ibandronate 6 mg also had lower bone pain scores and analgesic use. Treatment with ibandronate was well tolerated [18].

Oral ibandronate has been evaluated in phase III clinical trials of patients with bone metastases from breast cancer. In two pooled phase III studies, 564 patients with breast cancer and bone metastases were randomized to receive oral ibandronate 50 mg or placebo once daily for up to 96 weeks. The primary end point was again the SMPR, defined as the number of 12-week periods with new skeletal complications. Oral ibandronate significantly reduced the mean SMPR compared with placebo (0.95 vs. 1.18). There were also significant reductions in the mean number of events requiring radiotherapy (0.73 vs. 0.98) or surgery (0.47 vs. 0.53). The incidence of mild treatment-related nausea/vomiting was slightly higher in the ibandronate group than in the placebo group, but very few serious drug-related adverse events were reported [19].

The use of an oral agent is obviously attractive to both patients and health care providers but comparative data with other bisphosphonates are needed before a move away from intravenous treatment can be recommended.

A potential preventive effect of oral bisphosphonates was studied in retrospective analyses of large cohorts of women with osteoporosis. Interestingly, women who received bisphosphonates for osteoporosis had a 32% relative reduction in the overall risk of breast cancer compared with those who not receiving bisphosphonates. These correlations suggest that bisphosphonate-induced changes to the microenvironment surrounding potential cancer cells can prevent breast cancer. However, these results were generated from retrospective studies and in the absence of a prospective, randomized study of prevention [20, 21].

Gnant et al. investigated the effect of adding 3 years of zoledronic acid every 6 months to combination treatment either with tamoxifen and goserelin or with anastrozole and goserelin in 1803 premenopausal women with early, endocrine-responsive breast cancer [22]. The addition of zoledronic acid to endocrine therapy led to a relative reduction of 36% in the risk of disease progression compared with endocrine therapy alone and, although not significant, there was a trend toward improved overall survival. In addition, emerging evidence suggests that zoledronic acid has anti-tumor and anti-metastatic properties, including the inhibition of angiogenesis, tumor-cell invasion, adhesion in bone, and the induction of apoptosis [23].

A definite adjuvant role for bisphosphonates will require much larger randomized studies, such as the NSABP B34 study, with oral clodronate vs. placebo in 3300 patients with stage I–III breast cancer, or the AZURE trial, a large study of adjuvant zoledronic acid in 3360 patients with stage II/III breast cancer.

3.4 Prostate Cancer

Bone metastases develop in 65–75% of patients with metastatic prostate cancer [24]. The median overall survival for men with metastatic prostate cancer is 2–3 years. Approximately 50% of patients with bone metastases from prostate carcinoma will experience SREs during the course of the disease. In the metastatic setting, patients may experience multiple SREs, including pathological fractures, spinal cord compression, surgery, or radiotherapy to bone. Bone lesions from prostate carcinoma are typically osteoblastic in appearance.

Randomized, placebo-controlled trials of early-generation bisphosphonates (clodronate, elidronate, and pamidronate) failed to demonstrate a significant reduction in the frequency of skeletal complications in patients with bone metastases from prostate cancer [25]. Instead, zoledronic acid is the only bisphosphonate that has demonstrated objective long-term (2 year) efficacy in patients with bone metastases from prostate carcinoma and has achieved widespread regulatory approval in this setting.

Saad et al. [26] randomly assigned more than 600 patients with hormone-refractory prostate cancer and a history of bone metastases to a double-blind treatment regimen of intravenous zoledronic acid at 4 or 8 mg (subsequently reduced to 4 mg), or placebo every 3 weeks for 15 months. SREs were reported in a greater proportion of patients who received placebo than in those who received zoledronic acid at 4 mg (44.2 vs. 33.2%). Median time to first SRE was 321 days for patients who received placebo; it was not reached for patients who received zoledronic acid at 4 mg. Urinary markers of bone resorption were statistically significantly decreased in patients receiving zoledronic acid at either dose ($p = 0.001$). A greater increase in pain and analgesic scores was registered in patients receiving placebo than in those receiving zoledronic acid, but there were no differences in disease progression, performance status, or quality of life scores among the groups. Zoledronic acid at 4 mg given as a 15 min infusion was well tolerated, but the 8-mg dose was associated with deteriorations in renal function.

Bone loss induced by cancer treatment is a particularly important long-term problem for men receiving androgen deprivation therapy (ADT). The side effects of continuous ADT increase with the duration of treatment [27]. Bone mineral density of the hip and spine decreases by approximately 2–3% per year during initial therapy. Retrospective studies indicate a significantly increased fracture rate, with an estimated 10 year probability of fracture at around 40% with long-term use, compared to less than 20% in prostate cancer patients not receiving ADT [24]. Bisphosphonates have been used to prevent and treat bone loss in men with prostate cancer who are receiving ADT. Pamidronate (60 mg every 3 months) and alendronate significantly prevented bone mineral density loss compared to placebo in two separate trials involving men receiving ADT for non-metastatic prostate cancer [28, 29].

In a multi-center double-blind placebo-controlled clinical trial to assess the effect of zoledronic acid on bone mineral density during ADT for non-metastatic prostate cancer, Smith et al. randomized 106 men to receive 4 mg zoledronic acid or placebo intravenously every 3 months for 1 year. The primary efficacy variable was the percent change from baseline to 1 year in bone mineral density of the lumbar spine as measured by dual energy X-ray absorptiometry. Mean bone mineral density in the lumbar spine was found to have increased by 5.6% in men receiving zoledronic acid compared to a 2.2% decrease in those given placebo (mean difference 7.8%). Mean bone mineral density of the femoral neck, trochanter, and total hip also increased in the zoledronic acid group and decreased in the placebo group. Zoledronic acid was well tolerated [30].

Several more randomized controlled trials recently confirmed the efficacy of zoledronic acid (4 mg i.v. every 3 months for 1 year) compared to placebo in preventing bone mineral density loss at the lumbar spine and total hip in men with non-metastatic prostate cancer receiving ADT. The results were analyzed in a recent review [25].

3.5 Other Tumors: Lung, Kidney, Bladder and Thyroid

A significant proportion of patients with lung, kidney, bladder, and thyroid cancers develop bone metastases.

Rosen et al. previously reported the results of a phase III, multi-center, randomized, placebo-controlled trial that established the efficacy and safety of zoledronic acid in patients with bone metastases secondary to advanced lung carcinoma and other solid tumors [31]. After 9 months of treatment, zoledronic acid (given at a dose of 4 mg) significantly increased the time to first skeletal complication (median 230 days vs. 163 days for placebo), an important endpoint in this poor prognosis population, and significantly reduced the risk of developing SREs, as determined by multiple-event analysis (hazard ratio 0.732).

In another study [32], the long-term efficacy and safety results of this trial were reported after 21 months of continued therapy in patients with advanced carcinoma of the lung and other solid tumors. Patients treated with 4 mg of zoledronic acid experienced fewer skeletal complications, went significantly longer without experiencing a skeletal complication, and had a significantly lower risk than the placebo group of developing a skeletal complication. Zoledronic acid not only exhibited these effects at the time of therapy initiation but maintained consistent long-term benefits over the course of the 21 months of treatment. Most important, the long-term administration of 4 mg of zoledronic acid was well tolerated and the incidence of serious adverse events was similar to that in the placebo group.

In the study of Hatoum et al. [33], patients with solid tumors (including lung cancer) who were treated with zoledronic acid before the onset of skeletal complications had a 33% reduced risk of skeletal complications compared with patients who received treatment after experiencing the SRE. These data suggest not only that ZOL is effective at delaying the onset and reducing the risk of SREs, but also that early initiation and continuous treatment with bone-conserving therapy may increase the bone-related benefit in this patient population [34].

The natural history of bone metastases from renal cell carcinoma was evaluated recently by Zekri et al. in a 5 year review of 103 patients with metastatic renal cell carcinoma who were receiving standard therapy. Renal cell carcinoma patients with bone metastases were found to be at high risk of skeletal complications [35].

A subset analysis of the larger clinical trial carried out by Rosen et al. [31] was performed to determine the efficacy of zoledronic acid in renal cell carcinoma patients. Among the subset of 74 patients with renal cell carcinoma, 46 were treated with 4 mg of zoledronic acid or placebo. Significantly fewer patients treated with 4 mg zoledronic acid had a SRE (37 vs. 74% for placebo, $p = 0.015$), and zoledronic acid significantly prolonged the time to first SRE (median not reached at 9 months vs. 72 days for placebo; $p = 0.006$). Zoledronic acid significantly reduced the annual incidence of SREs by approximately 21% (mean 2.68 vs. 3.38 events per year for placebo, $p = 0.014$) and significantly reduced the risk of developing a SRE by 61% compared with placebo (risk ratio = 0.394, $p = 0.008$) by multiple event analysis. Median time to progression of bone lesions was also significantly extended with zoledronic acid treatment ($p = 0.014$) [36]. Thirteen patients with renal cell carcinoma were enrolled in the extension phase of this trial. The results from the 21 month extension phase confirmed and extended those of the 9 month study. Moreover, the median times to first event in the 4 mg zoledronic acid group were reached for SRE (median, 424 vs. 72 days for placebo) and bone lesion progression (median, 589 vs. 89 days for placebo), suggesting possible anti-tumor effects [32].

In the absence of a prospective randomized trial in patients with bone metastases from renal cell carcinoma, which is needed for definitive conclusions, this post-hoc subset analysis provides important insights into skeletal morbidity and treatment benefits in this setting.

Among the 773 patients enrolled in the phase III study of zoledronic acid in lung cancer and other solid tumors, 26 patients had bone metastases from bladder cancer. A retrospective subset analysis of patients with advanced bladder cancer revealed a reduced risk of any SRE with zoledronic acid compared to placebo (33 vs. 41%, respectively); however, small patient numbers precluded the results from being statistically significant [37].

Given the risk of skeletal events in thyroid cancer compared with other cancers bisphosphonates treatment should be employed also in patients with bone metastases from differentiated thyroid carcinoma (DTC). In one small study, DTC patients who had been administered pamidronate (90 mg, as a 2 h i.v. infusion monthly for 12 consecutive cycles) showed a significant decrease in bone pain, improved performance status, and improved quality of life. However, no significant decrease in analgesic consumption was recorded. A partial radiographic response of bone lesions was observed in two out of ten patients. Side effects were mild and transient [38]. The current practice is to use the same protocols as for breast or prostate cancer, but definitive studies in this area are warranted [39].

3.6 Conclusions

Bone metastases are very frequent events in the natural history of the more common tumors. They portend a short-term prognosis and negatively affect the quality of life of cancer patients. Palliation of symptoms, especially pain, remains the first aim of any therapeutic approach in the management of bone metastases, with a multi-disciplinary effort guaranteeing the best results.

The medical oncologist, radiation oncologist, and orthopedic surgeon must all be involved at different steps, but bisphosphonates are also an important component of the multi-disciplinary approach to the treatment of bone metastases. Bisphosphonates significantly reduce the incidence and frequency of skeletal complications in addition to providing substantial relief to patients suffering from bone pain. However, the optimal timing and duration of bisphosphonates therapy remain to be defined.

The potential role for bisphosphonates in the prevention of bone metastases and their role in improving survival are under current evaluation in clinical trials in solid tumors. At the same time, studies at the basic research level continue to elucidate the interactions that occur between tumor cells and the bone microenvironment, thereby identifying potential novel targets for future therapeutic interventions.

References

1. Coleman RE (2001) Metastatic bone disease: clinical features, pathophysiology and treatment strategies. Cancer Treat Rev 27:165–176
2. Mundy GR (1998) Myeloma bone disease. Eur J Cancer 34:246–251
3. Roodman GD (2004) Mechanisms of bone metastasis. N Engl J Med 350:1655–1664
4. Chirgwin JM, Guise TA (2000) Molecular mechanisms of tumor-bone interactions in osteolytic metastases. Crit Rev Eukaryot Gene Expr 10:159–178
5. Rogers MJ, Frith JC, Luckman SP et al (1999) Molecular mechanisms of action of bisphosphonates. Bone 24(S5):73–79
6. Roelofs AJ, Thompson K, Gordon S et al (2006) Molecular mechanisms of action of bisphosphonates: current status. Clin Cancer Res 12(20 Pt 2):6222s–6230s
7. Holen I, Coleman RE (2010) Bisphosphonates as treatment of bone metastases. Curr Pharm Des 16:1262–1271
8. Aapro M, Abrahamsson PA, Body JJ et al (2008) Guidance on the use of bisphosphonates in solid tumours: recommendations of an international expert panel. Ann Oncol 19:420–432

9. Gralow J, Tripathy D (2007) Managing metastatic bone pain: the role of bisphosphonates. J Pain Symptom Manage 33:462–472
10. Botteman M, Barghout V, Stephens J et al (2006) Cost effectiveness of bisphosphonates in the management of breast cancer patients with bone metastases. Ann Oncol 17:1072–1082
11. Paterson AH, Powles TJ, Kanis JA et al (1993) Double-blind controlled trial of oral clodronate in patients with bone metastases from breast cancer. J Clin Oncol 11:59–65
12. Conte PF, Mauriac L, Calabresi F et al (1996) Delay in progression of bone metastases treated with intravenous pamidronate: results from a multicentre randomised controlled trial. J Clin Oncol 14:2552–2559
13. Theriault RL, Lipton A, Hortobagyi GN et al (1999) Pamidronate reduces skeletal morbidity in women with advanced breast cancer and lytic bone lesions: a randomised, placebo-controlled trial. J Clin Oncol 17:846–854
14. Hortobagyi GN, Theriault RL, Porter L et al (1996) Efficacy of pamidronate in reducing skeletal complications in patients with breast cancer and lytic bone metastases. New Engl J Med 335:1785–1791
15. Kohno N, Aoqi K, Minami H et al (2005) Zoledronic acid significantly reduces skeletal complications compared with placebo in Japanese women with bone metastases from breast cancer: a randomized, placebo-controlled trial. J Clin Oncol 23:3314–3321
16. Rosen LS, Gordon D, Kaminski M et al (2001) Zoledronic acid versus pamidronate in the treatment of skeletal metastases in patients with breast cancer or osteolytic lesions of multiple myeloma: a phase III, double-blind, comparative trial. Cancer J 7:377–387
17. Rosen LS, Gordon D, Kaminski M et al (2003) Long term efficacy and safety of zoledronic acid compared with pamidronate disodium in treatment of skeletal complications in patients with advanced multiple myeloma or breast cancer: a randomized, double-blind, multicenter, comparative trial. Cancer 98:1735–1744
18. Body JJ, Diel IJ, Lichinitzer M et al (2004) Oral ibandronate reduces the risk of skeletal complications in breast cancer patients with metastatic bone disease: results from two randomised, placebo-controlled phase III studies. Br J Cancer 90:1133–1137
19. Body JJ, Diel IJ, Lichinitzer M et al (2003) Intravenous ibandronate reduces the incidence of skeletal complications in patients with breast cancer and bone metastases. Ann Oncol 14:1399–1405
20. Powles T, Paterson A, McCloskey E et al (2006) Reduction in bone relapse and improved survival with oral clodronate for adjuvant treatment of operable breast cancer [ISRCTN83688026]. Breast Cancer Res 8:R13
21. Chlebowski RT, Chen Z, Cauley J et al (2010) Oral bisphosphonate use and breast cancer incidence in postmenopausal women. J Clin Oncol 28(22):3582–3590
22. Gnant M, Mlineritsch B, Schippinger W et al (2009) Endocrine therapy plus zoledronic acid in premenopausal breast cancer. N Engl J Med 360:679–691
23. Daubine F, Le Gall C, Gasser J et al (2007) Antitumor effects of clinical dosing regimens of bisphosphonates in experimental breast cancer bone metastasis. J Natl Cancer Inst 99: 322–330
24. Allain TJ (2006) Prostate cancer, osteoporosis and fracture risk. Gerontology 52:107–110
25. Coleman R (2010) The use of bisphosphonates in cancer treatment Ann N Y Acad Sci. 28 Sept, DOI:10.1111/j.1749-6632.2010.05766.x
26. Saad F, Gleason DM, Murray R et al (2002) A randomized, placebo- controlled trial of zoledronic acid in patients with hormone-refractory metastatic prostate carcinoma. J Natl Cancer Inst 94:1458–1468
27. Preston DM, Torrens JI, Harding P et al (2002) Androgen deprivation in men with prostate cancer is associated with an increased rate of bone loss. Prostate Cancer Prostatic Dis 5:304–310
28. Bruder JM, Ma JZ, Wing N et al (2006) Effects of alendronate on bone mineral density in men with prostate cancer treated with androgen deprivation therapy. J Clin Densitom 9:431–437

29. Greenspan SL, Nelson JB, Trump DL et al (2007) Effect of once-weekly oral alendronate on bone loss in men receiving androgen deprivation therapy for prostate cancer: a randomized trial. Ann Intern Med 146:416–424
30. Smith MR, Eastham J, Gleason DM et al (2003) Randomized controlled trial of zoledronic acid to prevent bone loss in men receiving androgen deprivation therapy for non metastatic prostate cancer. J Urol 169:2008–2012
31. Rosen LS, Gordon D, Tchekmedyian S et al (2003) Zoledronic acid versus placebo in the treatment of skeletal metastases in patients with lung cancer and other solid tumors: a phase III, double-blind, randomized trial—the Zoledronic Acid Lung Cancer and Other Solid Tumors Study Group. J Clin Oncol 21:3150–3157
32. Rosen LS, Gordon D, Tchekmedyian S et al (2004) Long term efficacy and safety of zoledronic acid in the treatment of skeletal metastases in patients with non small cell lung carcinoma and other solid tumors: a randomized, Phase III, double-blind, placebo-controlled trial. Cancer 100:2613–2621
33. Hatoum HT, Lin SJ, Smith MR et al (2008) Zoledronic acid and skeletal complications in patients with solid tumors and bone metastases: analysis of a national medical claims database. Cancer 113:1438–1445
34. Langer C, Hirsh V (2010) Skeletal morbidity in lung cancer patients with bone metastases: demonstrating the need for early diagnosis and treatment with bisphosphonates. Lung Cancer 67:4–11
35. Zekri J, Ahmed N, Coleman RE et al (2001) The skeletal metastatic complications of renal cell carcinoma. Int J Oncol 19:379–382
36. Lipton A, Colombo-Berra A, Bukowski RM et al (2004) Skeletal complications in patients with bone metastases from renal cell carcinoma and therapeutic benefits of zoledronic acid. Clin Cancer Res 10:6397S–6403S
37. Mulders PFA, Miller K, Tchekmedyian NS et al. (2007) Long-term reduction in risk of skeletal complications with zoledronic acid in patients with advanced renal cell carcinoma or bladder cancer. Presented at: 22nd Annual EAU Congress; March 21; Berlin, Germany
38. Vitale G, Fonderico F, Martignetti A et al (2001) Pamidronate improves the quality of life and induces clinical remission of bone metastases in patients with thyroid cancer. Br J Cancer 84:1586–1590
39. Muresan MM, Olivier P, Leclere J et al (2008) Bone metastases from differentiated thyroid carcinoma. Endocr Relat Cancer 15:37–49

4 Use of Bisphosphonates in Hematology

Caterina Musolino and Alessandro Allegra

Abstract
Bisphosphonates (BPs) are used in the treatment of bone diseases associated with hematologic pathologies. BP therapy is, in fact, the mainstay of treatment for bone disease in multiple myeloma (MM) patients. These drugs decrease the frequency and delay the development of skeletal events in MM. Moreover BPs are used for the treatment of the malignancy-associated hypercalcemia seen in patients with blood diseases, such as MM and adult T-cell leukemia/lymphoma. Finally, an anti-tumor effect of BPs in MM patients has been described. However, BP-induced osteonecrosis of the jaw (BIONJ) is an unremitting adverse outcome. This chapter reviews the current theories explaining the mechanism for this complication. We report evidence for the use of BPs in hematologic diseases and provide recommendations to guide the clinical practice of treating bone disease in hematologic patients.

4.1 Introduction

Bisphosphonates (BPs) are a class of drugs developed over the past three decades for the treatment of metabolic bone diseases with high bone turnover, such as Paget's disease, tumor-associated osteolysis, and osteoporosis. The pharmacokinetic profile of BPs also makes them very suitable and safe drugs for the treatment of bone diseases in hematologic pathologies [1]. BP therapy is, in fact, the mainstay of treatment for bone disease related to multiple myeloma (MM);

C. Musolino (✉)
Division of Hematology, University of Messina, Messina, Italy
e-mail: cmusolino@unime.it

F. S. De Ponte (ed.), *Bisphosphonates and Osteonecrosis of the Jaw: A Multidisciplinary Approach*, DOI: 10.1007/978-88-470-2083-2_4,

it has decreased the frequency of skeletal events in MM and delayed their development [2].

Multiple myeloma is the second most common hematologic malignancy and the most common malignancy to involve bone, as more than 85% of patients with MM have bone involvement, which can be devastating. Approximately 45% of patients with MM experience a fracture in the first year after diagnosis, and 65% experience a fracture during the course of the disease [3, 4].

Advanced MM is accompanied by bone lesions resulting from the heightened osteolytic activity of osteoclasts and decreased rates of osteogenesis by osteoblasts. Therefore, patients with myeloma bone disease are at increased risk for skeletal-related events (SREs), such as pathologic fracture, the need for radiotherapy or surgery to bone, spinal cord compression, and hypercalcemia of malignancy. Each of these can reduce patients' functional independence, quality of life (QoL), and survival. Terpos et al. pointed out that high N-terminal cross-linked telopeptide of type I collagen was the only variable associated with an elevated risk of death [5]. Patients with MM who develop a pathological fracture were reported to have a greater than 20% increased risk of death [6].

Bone disease in MM patients may be due to several factors. Suppression of osteoblast precursor differentiation and induction of apoptosis in mature osteoblasts result in decreased bone formation. Increased production of molecules, such as dickkopf-1 and secreted frizzled-related protein 2, which act as Wingless-type signaling antagonists, are, at least in part, responsible for the osteoblast dysfunction in MM [7–9]. Other molecules, such as interleukin (IL)-7, IL-3, and transforming growth factor (TGF)-β, have been shown to inhibit osteoblastic differentiation in vitro [10–13]. Apoptosis of osteoblasts is mediated by the increased expression of the Fas ligand and tumor necrosis factor (TNF)-related apoptosis-inducing ligand on myeloma cells, which activate the Fas receptor and the death receptor on cells of the osteoblast lineage [14]. Furthermore, macrophage inflammatory protein 1-α, hepatocyte growth factor, and vascular endothelial growth factor (VEGF) are increased in the bone microenvironment, further stimulating osteoclastogenesis and bone digestion [15–19].

Bisphosphonates have been demonstrated to reduce the number of skeletal events, the need for radiation or surgery, and spinal cord compression. The reduction and control of pain is a crucial aspect in maintaining a high QoL in MM patients [20–22].

4.2 Adverse Effects of Bisphosphonates

Until a few years ago, BP therapy of MM was generally considered well tolerated and associated with minimal adverse effects [23]. These adverse effects can be separated into three groups: acute-phase reactions, upper aerodigestive tract issues, and effects concerning renal function [24]. In 2003, a fourth adverse effect, bisphosphonate-associated osteonecrosis of the jaw (BP-ONJ), was described for the first time [25] and has been diagnosed with increasing frequency. ONJ is a potentially serious complication of BPs. It is defined as the presence of exposed bone in the maxillofacial region that does not heal within 8 weeks after identification by a health care provider in a patient either receiving or with a history of exposure to a BP and who did not undergo radiation therapy to the craniofacial region [26–28].

4.2.1 Epidemiology and Pathogenesis

The incidence of BP-ONJ in MM patients is largely unknown; to date, only a few studies and one web-based survey have been published [29–35]. However the prevalence in all retrospective studies for MM ranges from 3 to 11% and in prospective studies from 7 to 21% [36].

How this process occurs is unclear but several theories have been advanced to explain the mechanism for BP-ONJ [37–39]. One theory suggests that it is caused by a cessation of bone remodeling and bone turnover due to the basic osteoclast-inhibiting effect of these drugs. After BP therapy, not enough osteoclasts can be activated to remove necrotic bone. A sufficient volume of necrotic bone results, which produces local changes sufficient to destroy the bony, vascular, and connective tissue structures necessary for self-repair [40].

Ardine et al. [41] reported that patients with BP-ONJ have persistently higher parathyroid hormone (PTH) levels than controls without ONJ and they suggested that high PTH is involved in BP-ONJ pathogenesis. Evidence against this theory is that in patients with primary hyperparathyroidism and elevated PTH, lesions in the oral cavity include reduced radicular lamina dura, reduced interdental alveolar bone density, and reduced cortical bone at the gonial index [42], whereas BP-ONJ is characterized by osteopetrosis-like osseous sclerosis with thickening of the lamina dura and of the alveolar crest and sclerosis of the alveolar margin [43].

A different theory is based on experimental evidence showing that pamidronate (PAM) and zoledronate (ZOL) inhibit capillary angiogenesis, decrease capillary tube formation, and inhibit endothelial growth factors and vessel sprouting, both in vitro and in a rat model [44].

Wood et al. have shown that BPs inhibit endothelial proliferation in cultured human umbilical vein and rat aortic ring cells. The same investigators demonstrated that ZOL is able to reduce vessel sprouting in the chicken-egg chorioallantoic membrane assay [45, 46].

Furthermore, a significant decrease of circulating VEGF levels was noted in patients receiving a single dose of PAM. The decrease in VEGF was already significant on day 1 after a single PAM infusion and the reduction persisted on day 7 [47]. Differently from PAM, ZOL induced a more prolonged decrease in serum VEGF levels, lasting 21 days from the time of infusion [49].

Moreover, in a study performed on MM patients, the administration of BPs was able to change soluble VEGF receptor 1 (sVEGFR1) concentrations, and MM patients without ONJ showed an increased level of sVEGFR1 after BP

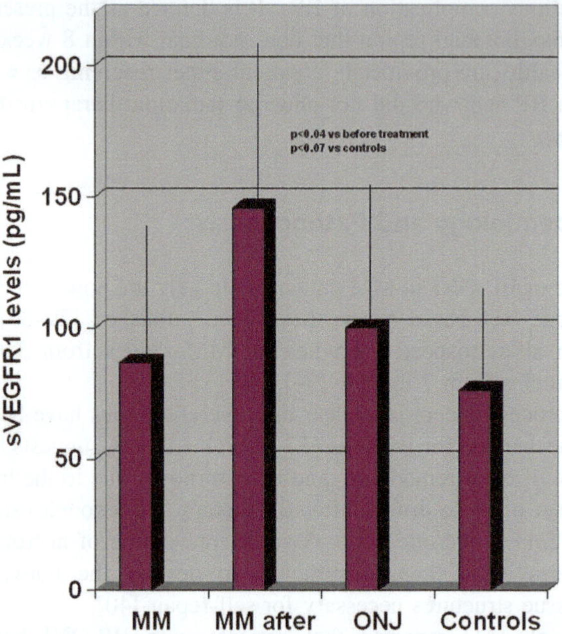

Fig. 4.1 Soluble vascular endothelial growth factor (sVEGFR1) levels in all groups studied. (From [50], ©2007 Informa Healthcare. Reproduced with permission)

administration (Fig. 4.1). However, in that study the authors were unable to detect a significant difference in sVEGFR1 between ONJ patients, MM patients before BP treatment, and control subjects [50].

Furthermore to test the hypothesis that in patients with ONJ there may be endothelial-cell interference by BPs, Allegra et al. used flow cytometry to evaluate the number of circulating endothelial cells (CECs). They characterized circulating endothelial progenitor cells (EPCs), which represent more immature cells, expressing the phenotype CD34+133+VEGFR2+. They also identified the more mature CECs, which lose CD133 and start to differentiate into mature endothelial cells. The phenotype of CECs thus is CD34+133-VEGFR2+. EPCs and CECs were found to be higher in MM patients than in either controls or ONJ patients. Moreover, ONJ patients had fewer EPCs than control subjects [51]. Analogous results were obtained by Ziebart et al., who showed that human umbilical vein endothelial cells and EPCs were significantly influenced by BPs at different concentrations compared with the non-treated control cells [52]. Taken together, these data suggest that in patients with ONJ, there is a suppressive effect of BPs on angiogenesis through an action on CECs. This finding is of potential interest because it is well known that in MM angiogenesis governs disease progression and that CECs are increased and vary in parallel with the clinical indicators of disease activity [53, 54].

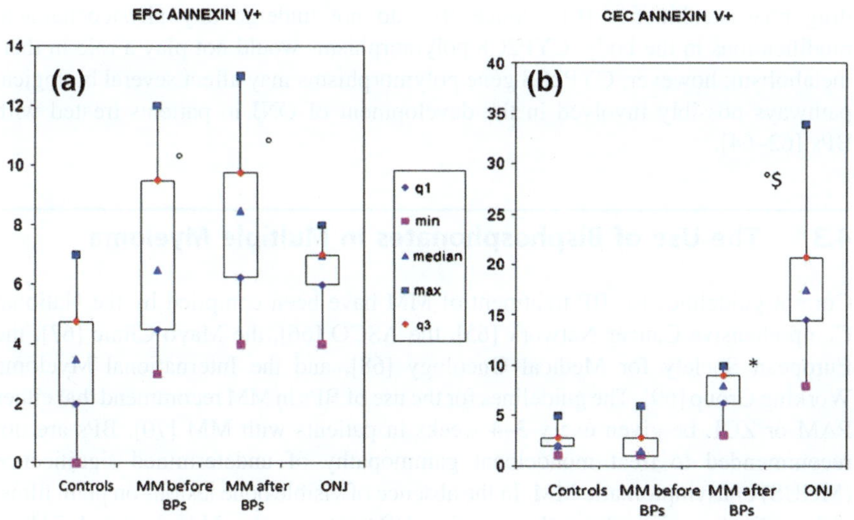

Fig. 4.2 Evaluation of endothelial progenitor cells (EPC) and annexin V+ circulating endothelial cells (CEC) cells in all groups. **a** # $p < 0.05$ vs. controls. Patients with osteonecrosis of the jaw (ONJ) had a higher percentage of EPC/annexin V+ cells (83%). **b** * $p < 0.05$ vs. controls and multiple myeloma (MM) patients before bisphosphonates (BPs); ° $p < 0.01$ vs. controls and MM patients before BPs; $ $p < 0.05$ vs. MM patients after BPs. (From [55] with permission by S. Karger AG, Basel)

Finally, an increase in endothelial cell apoptosis was demonstrated in MM patients after BP administration and in patients with ONJ (Fig. 4.2), with a correlation between the number of apoptotic cells and the duration of BP treatment in the latter group [55].

A recent case of bevacizumab-related ONJ highlights the potential of anti-angiogenic action to contribute to oral mucosal breakdown and suggests a cumulative toxicity between BPs and the anti-angiogenic agents commonly used in MM patients, such as thalidomide and lenalidomide [56, 57].

However, ONJ could be caused by a combination of environmental and genetic risk factors [58]. Sarasquete et al. explored the potential role of genetics in the development of ONJ in MM patients under BP therapy. A genome-wide association study was performed analyzing 500,568 single nucleotide polymorphisms (SNPs) in two series of homogeneously treated MM patients, one with and the other without ONJ. Four SNPs that mapped within the cytochrome P450-2C gene (CYP2C8) showed a different distribution between cases and controls, with statistically significant differences. SNP rs1934951 was significantly associated with a higher risk of ONJ development. Genotyping results identified an over-representation of the T allele in cases compared with controls (48 vs. 12%). Thus, individuals homozygous for the T allele had an increased likelihood of developing ONJ [59]. CYP2C8 is responsible for the metabolism of several drugs [60], and recent reports have shown that variability in genes encoding CYP2C8 may affect drug pharmacokinetics [61]. Since BPs do not undergo any physicochemical modifications in the body, CYP2C8 polymorphisms would not play a role in their metabolism; however, CYP2C8 gene polymorphisms may affect several biological pathways possibly involved in the development of ONJ in patients treated with BPs [62–64].

4.3 The Use of Bisphosphonates in Multiple Myeloma

Current guidelines for BP treatment of MM have been compiled by the National Comprehensive Cancer Network [65], the ASCO [66], the Mayo Clinic [67], the European Society for Medical Oncology [68], and the International Myeloma Working Group [69]. The guidelines for the use of BPs in MM recommend that either PAM or ZOL be given every 3–4 weeks in patients with MM [70]. BPs are not recommended to treat monoclonal gammopathy of undetermined significance (MGUS) or asymptomatic MM. In the absence of visible bone lesions on plain films, if the patient requires chemotherapy, then BP treatment should be initiated [71].

BPs should be given for 2 years and after that at the physician's discretion, with therapy resumed upon relapse. While the administration of BPs beyond 2 years is not recommended, a subgroup of patients might still benefit from longer treatment. As an alternative to stopping BPs after 2 years, some panel members prefer to continue BP therapy at either a reduced dose or a reduced schedule.

Cafro et al. evaluated the incidence, risk factors, management, and prevention strategies of ONJ in order to optimize the current standard use of BPs in MM. The most important risk factor for ONJ was determined to be the number of BPs infusions [72]. Additional risk factors in cancer patients include the underlying malignancy, chemotherapy, corticosteroids, and systemic or regional infection. Pancytopenia secondary to cancer and/or cancer treatment is a risk for infection and osteomyelitis. Vascular insufficiency due to thrombosis caused by coagulopathies also has been associated with ONJ [73]. Other risk factors are diabetes, smoking, alcohol use, and poor oral hygiene [74]. Nonetheless, the major risk factors for ONJ remain duration of treatment with BPs, the type and dosage of BP used, and dental procedures/trauma [75–79]. The risk for ONJ increases with BP treatment duration and has been shown to be 5–15% at 4 years [80–87].

A retrospective study of MM patients treated with ZOL on a reduced schedule (infusion every 3 months vs. monthly) showed a decrease in the number of ONJ cases [88]. While ONJ has been reported in patients treated with the oral BP clodronate, such cases are very uncommon [89].

In agreement with the guidelines, a prevention-based strategy was recommended by the panels of experts. Specifically, as the majority of ONJ cases occur after dental surgery [90–92], MM patients should receive a comprehensive dental examination before treatment with BPs, in order to identify and treat dental problems that may require surgical or invasive dental procedures. After therapy initiation, unnecessary invasive dental procedures should be avoided.

Montefusco et al. analyzed the data of 178 patients with MM to evaluate whether antibiotic prophylaxis before dental procedures can prevent ONJ. The only variable significantly associated with ONJ was antibiotic prophylaxis, which had a protective effect [93].

Established ONJ should be managed conservatively; a BP "drug holiday" is usually indicated and invasive surgery should generally be avoided [94].

4.4 Bisphosphonates and Hematology: Not Only Multiple Myeloma

4.4.1 Bisphosphonates and Hematopoietic Cell Transplantation

Although BPs are frequently used in the treatment of MM patients, there are other hematologic conditions in which BPS might be used.

Long-term survivors of hematopoietic cell transplantation (HCT) are at risk for loss of bone mineral density (BMD) and subsequent osteoporosis. Bone loss occurs predominantly within the first 6–12 months after autologous and allogeneic HCT. Recovery first occurs in the lumbar spine and is followed by a slower recovery of BMD in the femoral neck. BMD may not return to baseline levels in patients with continuing exposure to corticosteroids and calcineurin inhibitors. There is a lack of clear guidelines for the screening, prevention, and treatment of bone loss after HCT. However, general interventions to reduce fracture risk, including adequate intake of calcium and vitamin D, are advised for all HCT recipients; where indicated, BPs can be used for the prevention or treatment of osteoporosis in adult HCT recipients [95].

Grade 2–4 acute graft versus host disease (GVHD) is associated with bone loss at 1 year after stem cell transplantation, whereas extensive chronic GVHD and steroid use are unfavorable prognostic factors in terms of osteopenia/osteoporosis at 2 years post-transplantation. The use of ZOL significantly prevented bone loss in the femoral neck and in the spine [96].

4.4.2 Bisphosphonate and Hypercalcemia

Hypercalcemia is a common metabolic complication of malignant disease and often requires emergency intervention. Although it is more frequently associated with solid tumors, malignancy-associated hypercalcemia (MAH) is seen in a significant number of patients with blood diseases, and its association with myeloma and adult T-cell leukemia/lymphoma is well recognized. BPs have revolutionized the management of MAH over the last 20 years [97]. They are also safely used in treating childhood hypercalcemia, secondary to acute lymphocytic leukemia [98, 99].

4.5 Anti-tumor Effects of Bisphosphonates in Multiple Myeloma

The option to use BPs in the treatment of MM recently received a new impulse by data showing that ZOL and PAM may have synergistic or additive effects with MM therapy and, in the future, might successfully be used in conjunction with other anti-myeloma agents. ZOL has been shown to decrease bone tumor burden in an established MM animal model [100–102], while PAM has also shown anti-myeloma activity in animal models in vivo [103, 104].

Amino-bisphosphonates exert their anti-neoplastic effects by several mechanisms. It is well established that they inhibit the mevalonate pathway, thereby affecting cell function and survival duration. Nitrogen-containing bisphosphonates also have been shown to directly induce tumor apoptosis and inhibit angiogenesis, in addition to their actions on the immune system and osteoblasts [105–107].

To study the inhibitory effect of ZOL on the growth and CD138 expression of myeloma cell line KM3, Hou et al. treated the cells with different concentrations of ZOL. The results showed that ZOL inhibited the growth of KM3 cells in a dose-dependent manner [108].

Moreover BPs induce significant expansion of $\gamma\delta$-T cells. In a study by Abe et al. ZOL-activated $V\gamma9\gamma\delta$T-lymphocyte-activated killer cells were administered to patients with MM. The results suggested that this strategy could be a safe and promising immunotherapy for the treatment of patients with MM [109].

4.6 Conclusions

The positive impact of BPs on the management of millions of patients with bone disorders has been enormous. These drugs have a pivotal role in the treatment of patients with malignant diseases involving bone, and thus a potentially enormous impact on the cost of disease treatment. In the USA, the national cost burden for patients with metastatic bone disease in 2004 dollars was estimated at $12.6 billion in total direct medical costs. In a recent study, 5.3% of cancer patients in the USA were projected to have metastatic bone disease. Hematologic disease was the leading cause, with MM accounting for 28.8% of these cases [110].

Currently, MM patients cannot be successfully managed without BPs. The recognition of ONJ as a late toxicity complication of BP treatment and the recent advances in basic and clinical research regarding the effects of BP therapy in the pathobiology of MM warrant an update in therapeutic strategies to redefine the balance between the risks and benefits of this class of drugs.

References

1. Holmberg AR, Lerner UH, Alayia AA et al (2010) Development of a novel poly bisphosphonate conjugate for treatment of skeletal metastasis and osteoporosis. J Oncol 37(3):563–567
2. Levy J, Roodman GD (2009) The role of bisphosphonates in multiple myeloma. Curr Hematol Malig Rep 4(2):108–112
3. Melton LJ 3rd, Kyle RA, Achenbach SJ et al (2005) Fracture risk with multiple myeloma: a population based study. J Bone Miner Res 20:487–493
4. Mahnken AH, Wildberger JE, Gehbauer G et al (2002) Multidetector CT of the spine in multiple myeloma: comparison with MR imaging and radiography. AJR 178:1429–1436
5. Terpos E, Berenson J, Cook RJ et al (2010) Prognostic variables for survival and skeletal complications in patients with multiple myeloma osteolytic bone disease. Leukemia 24(5):1043–1049
6. Saad F, Lipton A, Cook R et al (2007) Pathological fractures correlate with reduced survival in patients with malignant bone disease. Cancer 110:1860–1867
7. Silvestris F, Cafforio P, Calvani N et al (2004) Impaired osteoblastogenesis in myeloma bone disease: role of upregulated apoptosis by cytokines and malignant plasma cells. Br J Haematol 126(4):475–486
8. Tian E, Zhan F, Walker R et al (2003) The role of the Wnt-signaling antagonist DKK1 in the development of osteolytic lesions in multiple myeloma. N Engl J Med 349(26):2483–2494
9. Oshima T, Abe M, Asano J et al (2005) Myeloma cells suppress bone formation by secreting a soluble Wnt inhibitor, sFRP-2. Blood 106(9):3160–3165
10. Giuliani N, Colla S, Morandi F et al (2005) Myeloma cells block RUNX2/CBFA1 activity in human bone marrow osteoblast progenitors and inhibit osteoblast formation and differentiation. Blood 106(7):2472–2483
11. Ehrlich LA, Chung HY, Ghobrial I et al (2005) IL-3 is a potential inhibitor of osteoblast differentiation in multiple myeloma. Blood 106(4):1407–1414
12. Franchimont N, Rydziel S, Canalis E (2000) Transforming growth factor-beta increases interleukin-6 transcripts in osteoblasts. Bone 26(3):249–253
13. Hayashi T, Hideshima T, Nguyen AN et al (2004) Transforming growth factor beta receptor I kinase inhibitor down-regulates cytokine secretion and multiple myeloma cell growth in the bone marrow microenvironment. Clin Cancer Res 10(22):7540–7546
14. Silvestris F, Cafforio P, Tucci M et al (2003) Upregulation of osteoblast apoptosis by malignant plasma cells: a role in myeloma bone disease. Br J Haematol 122(1):39–52
15. Sati HIA, Greaves M, Apperley JF et al (1999) Expression of interleukin-1b and tumour necrosis factor-alpha in plasma cells from patients with multiple myeloma. Br J Haematol 104(2):350–357
16. Roux S, Mariette X (2004) The high rate of bone resorption in multiple myeloma is due to RANK (receptor activator of nuclear factor-Kb) and RANK ligand expression. Leuk Lymphoma 45(6):1111–1118
17. Oyajobi BO, Mundy GR (2003) Receptor activator of NF-kappaB ligand, macrophage inflammatory protein-1alpha, and the proteasome: novel therapeutic targets in myeloma. Cancer 97(3):813–817
18. Mitsiades CS, Mitsiades N, Hideshima T et al (2006) Proteasome inhibition as a new therapeutic principle in hematological malignancies. Curr Drug Targets 7(10):1341–1347
19. Tanaka Y, Abe M, Hiasa M et al (2007) Myeloma cell-osteoclast interaction enhances angiogenesis together with bone resorption: a role for vascular endothelial cell growth factor and osteopontin. Clin Cancer Res 13(3):816–823
20. Vogel CL, Yanagihara RH, Wood AJ et al (2004) Safety and pain palliation of zoledronic acid in patients with breast cancer, prostate cancer, or multiple myeloma who previously received bisphosphonate therapy. Oncologist 9(6):687–695

21. Gralow J, Tripathy D (2007) Managing metastatic bone pain: the role of bisphosphonates. J Pain Symptom Manage 33(4):462–472
22. Ludwig H, Zojer N (2007) Supportive care in multiple myeloma. Best Pract Res Clin Haematol. 20(4):817–835
23. Dunstan C, Felsenberg D, Seibel MJ (2006) Therapy insight: the risks and benefits of bisphosphonates for the treatment of tumor-induced bone disease. Nat Clin Pract Oncol 4(1):42–55
24. Diel IJ, Bergner R, Grotz KA (2007) Adverse effects of bisphosphonates: current issues. J Support Oncol 5:475–482
25. Marx RE (2003) Pamidronate (Aredia) and zoledronate (Zometa) induced avascular necrosis of jaws: a growing epidemic. J Oral Maxillofac Surg 61:1115–1117
26. Walter C, Grotz KA, Kunkel M et al (2007) Prevalence of bisphosphonate associated osteonecrosis of the jaw within the field of osteonecrosis. Support Care Cancer 15: 197–202
27. Nastro E, Musolino C, Allegra A et al (2007) Bisphosphonate-associated osteonecrosis of the jaw in patients with multiple myeloma and breast cancer. Acta Haematol 117:181–187
28. Nastro E, Allegra A, Oteri G et al (2009) Avascular necrosis of bone in leukemia and osteonecrosis of jaw by bisphosphonate. J Oral Maxillofac Surg 67(12):2701–2703
29. Badros A, Weikel D, Salama A et al (2006) Osteonecrosis of the jaw in multiple myeloma patients: clinical features and risk factors. J Clin Oncol 24:945–952
30. Calvo-Villas JM, Tapia Torres M, Govantes Rodríguez J et al (2006) Osteonecrosis of the jaw in patients with multiple myeloma during and after treatment with zoledronic acid. Med Clin (Barc) 127:576–579
31. Dimopoulos MA, Kastritis E, Anagnostopoulos A et al (2006) Osteonecrosis of the jaw in patients with multiple myeloma treated with bisphosphonates: evidence of increased risk after treatment with zoledronic acid. Haematologica 91:968–971
32. Tosi P, Zamagni E, Cangini D et al (2006) Osteonecrosis of the jaws in newly diagnosed multiple myeloma patients treated with zoledronic acid and thalidomide-dexamethasone. Blood 108:3951–3952
33. Zervas K, Verrou E, Teleioudis Z et al (2006) Incidence, risk factors and management of osteonecrosis of the jaw in patients with multiple myeloma: a single-centre experience in 303 patients. Br J Haematol 134:620–623
34. Corso A, Varettoni M, Zappasodi P et al (2007) A different schedule of zoledronic acid can reduce the risk of the osteonecrosis of the jaw in patients with multiple myeloma. Leukemia 21:1545–1548
35. Petrucci MT, Gallucci C, Agrillo A et al (2007) Role of ozone therapy in the treatment of osteonecrosis of the jaws in multiple myeloma patients. Haematologica 92:1289–1290
36. Walter C, Al-Nawas B, Frickhofen N et al (2010) Prevalence of bisphosphonate associated osteonecrosis of the jaws in multiple myeloma patients. Head Face Med 6:11
37. Woo SB, Hellstein JW, Kalmar JR (2006) Narrative review: bisphosphonates and osteonecrosis of the jaws. Ann Intern Med 144:753–761
38. Van den Wyngaert T, Huizing MT, Vermorken JB (2007) Osteonecrosis of the jaw related to the use of bisphosphonates. Curr Opin Oncol 19:315–322
39. Mehrotra B, Ruggiero S (2006) Bisphosphonate complications including osteonecrosis of the jaw. Hematology 2006:356–360
40. Helstein JW, Cindy MS, Cindy L et al (2005) Bisphosphonate osteochemonecrosis (bis-phossy jaw): is this phossy jaw of the 21st century? J Oral Maxillofac Surg 63: 682–689
41. Ardine M, Generali D, Donadio M (2006) Could the long-term persistence of low serum calcium levels and high serum parathyroid hormone levels during bisphosphonate treatment predispose metastatic breast cancer patients to undergo osteonecrosis of the jaw? Ann Oncol 17:1336–1337

42. Padbury AD Jr, Tözüm TF, Taba M Jr et al (2006) The impact of primary hyperparathyroidism on the oral cavity. J Clin Endocrinol Metab 91:3439–3445
43. Phal PM, Myall RWT, Assael LA et al (2007) Imaging findings of bisphosphonate-associated osteonecrosis of the jaw. Am J Neuroradiol 28:1139–1145
44. Fournier P, Boissier S, Filleur S et al (2002) bisphosphonates inhibit angiogenesis in vitro and testosterone-stimulated vascular regrowth in the ventral prostate in castrated rats. Cancer Res 62:6538–6544
45. Wood J, Bonjean K, Ruetz S et al (2002) Novel antiangiogenic effects of the bisphosphonate compound zoledronic acid. J Pharmacol Exp Ther 302:1055–1061
46. Wood J, Schnell C, Green JR (2000) Zoledronic acid, a potent inhibitor of bone resorption, inhibits proliferation and induces apoptosis in human endothelial cells in vitro and is anti-angiogenic in a murine growth factor implant model. Proc Am Soc Clin Oncol 665:664–665
47. Santini D, Vincenzi B, Avvisati G et al (2002) Pamidronate induces modifications of circulating angiogenic factors in cancer patients. Clin Cancer Res 8:1080–1084
48. Vincenzi B, Santini D, Rocci L et al (2003) Bisphosphonates: new antiangiogenic molecules in cancer treatment? Ann Oncol 14:806–807
49. Ferretti G, Fabi A, Carlini P et al (2005) Zoledronic-acid-induced circulating level modifications of angiogenic factors, metalloproteinases and proinflammatory cytokines in metastatic breast cancer patients. Oncology 69:35–43
50. Alonci A, Allegra A, Bellomo G et al (2007) Patients with bisphosphonate-associated osteonecrosis of the jaw have unmodified levels of soluble vascular endothelial growth factor receptor 1. Leuk Lymphoma 48(9):1852–1854
51. Allegra A, Oteri G, Nastro E et al (2007) Patients with bisphosphonates-associated osteonecrosis of the jaw have reduced circulating endothelial cells. Hematol Oncol 25:164–169
52. Ziebart T, Pabst A, Klein MO et al (2011) Bisphosphonates: restrictions for vasculogenesis and angiogenesis: inhibition of cell function of endothelial progenitor cells and mature endothelial cells in vitro. Clin Oral Invest 15:105–111
53. Pruneti G, Ponzoni M, Ferreri A et al (2002) Microvessel density, a surrogate marker of angiogenesis, is significantly related to serviva in multiple myeloma patients. Br J Haematol 118:817–820
54. Zhang H, Vakil V, Braunstein M et al (2005) Circulating endothelial progenitor cells in multiple myeloma: implication and significance. Blood 105:3286–3294
55. Allegra A, Alonci A, Penna G et al (2010) Bisphosphonate induce apoptosis of circulating endothelial cells in multiple myeloma patients and in subjects with Bisphosphonate-induced Osteonecrosis of the jaws. Acta Haematol 124(2):79–85
56. Estilo CL, Fornier M, Farooki A et al (2008) Osteonecrosis of the jaw related to bevacizumab. J Clin Oncol 26(24):4037–4038
57. Ayllon J, Launay-Vacher V, Medioni J et al (2009) Osteonecrosis of the jaw under bisphosphonate and antiangiogenic therapies: cumulative toxicity profile? Ann Oncol 20(3):600–601
58. Walker BA, Leone PE, Jenner MW et al (2006) Integration of global SNP-based mapping and expression arrays reveals key regions, mechanisms, and genes important in the pathogenesis of multiple myeloma. Blood 108:1733–1743
59. Sarasquete ME, Garcıa-Sanz R, Marın L et al (2008) Bisphosphonate-related osteonecrosis of the jaw is associated with polymorphisms of the cytochrome P450 CYP2C8 in multiple myeloma: a genome-wide single nucleotide polymorphism analysis. Blood 112:2709–2712
60. Ingelman-Sundberg M, Sim SC, Gomez A et al (2007) Influence of cytochrome P450 polymorphisms on drug therapies: pharmacogenetic, pharmacoepigenetic and clinical aspects. Pharmacol Ther 116:496–526
61. Human Cytochrome P450 (CYP) Allele Nomenclature Committee. CYP2C8 allele nomenclature. http://www.cypalleles.ki.se/cyp2c8.htm. Accessed 11 May 2008

62. Fleming I (2007) Epoxyeicosatrienoic acids, cell signaling and angiogenesis. Prostaglandins Other Lipid Mediat 82:60–67
63. Capdevila JH, Falck JR, Harris RC (2000) Cytochrome P450 and arachidonic acid bioactivation. Molecular and functional properties of the arachidonate monooxygenase. J Lipid Res 41:163–181
64. Luckman SP, Hughes DE, Coxon FP et al (1998) Nitrogen-containing bisphosphonates inhibit the mevalonate pathway and prevent posttranslational prenylation of GTP-binding proteins, including Ras. J Bone Miner Res 13:581–589
65. Anderson K, Alsina M, Bensinger W et al (2007) National Comprehensive Cancer Network (NCCN). Multiple myeloma guidelines. J Natl Compr Canc Netw 5:118
66. Kyle RA, Yee GC, Somerfield MR et al (2007) American Society of Clinical Oncology 2007 clinical practice guideline update on the role of bisphosphonates in multiple myeloma. J Clin Oncol 25(17):2464–2472
67. Lacy MQ, Dispenzieri A, Gertz MA et al (2006) Mayo clinic consensus statement for the use of bisphosphonates in multiple myeloma. Mayo Clin Proc 81(8):1047–1053
68. Harrouseau JL, Greil R, Kloke O (2005) ESMO minimum clinical recommendations for diagnosis, treatment and follow-up of multiple myeloma. Ann Oncol 16(1):i45–i47
69. Durie BG (2007) Use of bisphosphonates in multiple myeloma: IMWG response to Mayo Clinic consensus statement. Mayo Clin Proc 82(4):516–517
70. Chern B, Joseph D, Joshua D et al (2004) Bisphosphonate infusions: patient preference, safety and clinic use. Support Care Cancer 12(6):463–466
71. Terpos E, Sezer P, Garcia-Sanz et al (2009) The use of bisphosphonates in multiple myeloma: recommendations o fan expert panel on behalf of the European Myeloma Network. Ann Oncol 20(8):1303–1317
72. Cafro AM, Barbarano L, Nosari AM et al (2008) Osteonecrosis of the jaw in patients with multiple myeloma treated with bisphosphonates: definition and management of the risk related to zoledronic acid. Clin Lymphoma Myeloma 8(2):111–116
73. Ruggiero S, Gralow J, Marx RE (2006) Practical guidelines for the prevention, diagnosis, and treatment of osteonecrosis of the jaw in patients with cancer. J Oncol Pract 2:7–14
74. American Association of Oral and Maxillofacial Surgeons Position Paper on Bisphosphonate-Related Osteonecrosis of the Jaws, September 25, 2006 http://www.aaoms.org/docs/position_papers/osteonecrosis.pdf
75. Hansen T, Kunkel M, Weber A, James Kirkpatrick C (2006) Osteonecrosis of the jaws in patients treated with bisphosphonates—histomorphologic analysis in comparison with infected osteoradionecrosis. J Oral Pathol Med 35(3):155–160
76. Weitzman R, Sauter N, Eriksen EF et al (2007) Critical review: updated recommendations for the prevention, diagnosis, treatment of osteonecrosis of the jaw in cancer patients—May 2006. Crit Rev Oncol Hematol 62(2):148–152
77. Bamias A, Kastritis E, Bamia C et al (2005) Osteonecrosis of the jaw in cancer after treatment with bisphosphonates: incidence and risk factors. J Clin Oncol 23(34):8580–8587
78. Melo MD, Obeid G (2005) Osteonecrosis of the jaws in patients with a history of receiving bisphosphonate therapy: strategies for prevention and early recognition. J Am Dent Assoc 136(12):1675–1681
79. Ruggiero SL, Mehrotra B, Rosenberg TJ et al (2004) Osteonecrosis of the jaws associated with the use of bisphosphonates: a review of 63 cases. J Oral Maxillofac Surg 62(5):527–534
80. Dimopoulos MA, Kastritis E, Anagnostopoulos A et al (2006) Osteonecrosis of the jaw in patients with multiple myeloma treated with bisphosphonates: evidence of increased risk after treatment with zoledronic acid. Haematologica 91(7):968–971
81. Zervas K, Verrou E, Teleioudis Z et al (2006) Incidence, risk factors and management of osteonecrosis of the jaw in patients with multiple myeloma: a single-centre experience in 303 patients. Br J Haematol 134(6):620–623
82. Durie BG, Katz M, Crowley J (2005) Osteonecrosis of the jaw and bisphosphonates. N Engl J Med 353(1):99–102

83. Mehrotra B, Ruggiero S (2006) Bisphosphonate complications including osteonecrosis of the jaw. Hematology Am Soc Hematol Educ Program 356-360
84. Montazeri AH, Erskine JG, McQuaker IG (2007) Oral sodium clodronate induced osteonecrosis of the jaw in a patient with myeloma. Eur J Haematol 79(1):69–71
85. Brooks JK, Gilson AJ, Sindler AJ et al (2007) Osteonecrosis of the jaws associated with use of risedronate: report of 2 new cases. Oral Surg Oral Med Oral Pathol Oral Radiol Endod 103(6):780–786
86. Yarom N, Yahalom R, Shoshani Y et al (2007) Osteonecrosis of the jaw induced by orally administered bisphosphonates: incidence, clinical features, predisposing factors and treatment outcome. Osteoporos Int 18(10):1363–1370
87. Mavrokokki T, Cheng A, Stein B et al (2007) Nature and frequency of bisphosphonate-associated osteonecrosis of the jaws in Australia. J Oral Maxillofac Surg 65(3):415–423
88. Corso A, Varettoni M, Zappasodi P et al (2007) A different schedule of zoledronic acid can reduce the risk of the osteonecrosis of the jaw in patients with multiple myeloma. Leukemia 21(7):1545–1548
89. Adam Z, Kozumplikova M, Pour L et al (2006) Osteonecrosis of the jaw in the course of multiple myeloma treatment and bisphosphonate administration. Vnitr Lek 52(2):176–180
90. Badros A, Terpos E, Katodritou E et al (2008) Natural history of osteonecrosis of the jaw in patients with multiple myeloma. J Clin Oncol 26(36):5904–5909
91. Coleman RE, Major P, Lipton A et al (2005) Predictive value of bone resorption and formation markers in cancer patients with bone metastases receiving the bisphosphonate zoledronic acid. J Clin Oncol 23(22):4925–4935
92. Attal M, Harousseau JL, Leyvraz S et al (2006) Maintenance therapy with thalidomide improves survival in patients with multiple myeloma. Blood 108(10):3289–3294
93. Montefusco V, Gay F, Spina F et al (2008) Antibiotic prophylaxis before dental procedures may reduce the incidence of osteonecrosis of the jaw in patients with multiple myeloma treated with bisphosphonates. Leuk Lymphoma 49(11):2156–2162
94. Dickinson M, Prince HM, Kirsa S et al (2009) Osteonecrosis of the jaw complicating bisphosphonate treatment for bone disease in multiple myeloma: an overview with recommendations for prevention and treatment. Intern Med J 39(5):304–316
95. McClune BL, Polgreen LE, Burmeister LA et al (2010) Screening, prevention and management of osteoporosis and bone loss in adult and pediatric hematopoietic cell transplant recipients. Bone Marrow Transplant. Aug 23. [Epub ahead of print]
96. Chae YS, Kim JG, Moon JH et al (2009) Pilot study on the use of zoledronic acid to prevent bone loss in allo-SCT recipients. Bone Marrow Transplant 44(1):35–41
97. Sargent JT, Smith OP (2010) Haematological emergencies managing hypercalcaemia in adults and children with haematological disorders. Br J Haematol 149(4):465–477
98. Schmid I, Stachel D, Schön C et al (2001) Pamidronate and calcitonin as therapy of acute cancer-related hypercalcemia in children. Klinische Padiatrie 213(1):30–34
99. Goldbloom EB, Cummings EA, Yhap M (2005) Osteoporosis at presentation of childhood ALL: management with pamidronate. Pediatr Hematol Oncol 22(7):543–550
100. Yaccoby S, Pearse RN, Johnson CL et al (2002) Myeloma interacts with the bone marrow microenvironment to induce osteoclastogenesis and is dependent on osteoclast activity. Br J Haematol 116(2):278–290
101. Yaccoby S, Wezeman MJ, Zangari M et al (2006) Inhibitory effects of osteoblasts and increased bone formation on myeloma in novel culture systems and a myelomatous mouse model. Haematologica 91(2):192–199
102. Croucher PI, De Hendrik R, Perry MJ et al (2003) Zoledronic acid treatment of 5T2MM-bearing mice inhibits the development of myeloma bone disease: evidence for decreased osteolysis, tumor burden and angiogenesis, and increased survival. J Bone Miner Res 18(3):482–492
103. Dhodapkar MV, Singh J, Mehta J et al (1998) Anti-myeloma activity of pamidronate in vivo. Br J Haematol 103(2):530–532

104. Kondo H, Mori A (2002) Anti-tumor activity of pamidronate in human multiple myeloma. Leuk Lymphoma 43(4):919–921
105. Santini D, Virzi V, Fratto ME et al (2010) Can we consider zoledronic acid a new antitumor agent? Recent evidence in clinical setting. Curr Cancer Drug Targets 10(1):46–54
106. Koizumi M, Nakaseko C, Ohwada C et al (2007) Zoledronate has an antitumor effect and induces actin rearrangement in dexamethasone-resistant myeloma cells. Eur J Haematol 79(5):382–391
107. Guenther A, Gordon S, Tiemann M et al (2010) The bisphosphonate zoledronic acid has antimyeloma activity in vivo by inhibition of protein prenylation. Int J Cancer 126(1): 239–246
108. Huang HM, Ding RS, Xiang XX, Hou J (2009) Effect of zoledronic acid on the growth and CD138 expression of myeloma cell line KM3. Zhonghua Xue Ye Xue Za Zhi 30(3): 183–185
109. Abe Y, Muto M, Nieda M et al (2009) Clinical and immunological evaluation of zoledronate-activated Vgamma9gammadelta T-cell-based immunotherapy for patients with multiple myeloma. Exp Hematol 37(8):956–968
110. Schulman KL, Kohles J (2007) Economic burden of metastatic bone disease in the U. S. Cancer 109:2334–2342

Use of Bisphosphonates in Osteoporosis

5

Angelina De Sarro and Letteria Minutoli

Abstract

Osteoporosis is the most common bone disease in humans and it can affect people of all ethnic backgrounds, especially older women and men. In osteoporosis, the low bone mass and microarchitectural deterioration of bone tissue lead to enhanced bone fragility and an increased susceptibility to fractures. The process of repair occurs in bone remodeling, which lasts about 6 months. The most common form of osteoporosis, experienced by postmenopausal women, results from reduced estrogen production, which disrupts the fine balance of the bone remodeling cycle as well as bone resorption. Bisphosphonates (BPs) have been the principal anti-resorptive agents used in the therapy of osteoporosis and they work because of two key properties: (1) strong binding to bone due to a high affinity for hydroxyapatite and (2) their ability to inhibit osteoclast function by inhibiting the enzyme farnesyl-diphosphate synthase. The major treatment goal for patients with osteoporosis is to prevent fractures by maintaining or increasing bone mineral density and reducing excessive bone turnover. Bisphosphonates are well tolerated, but, in many cases oral dosing options have failed because some patients suffer severe upper gastrointestinal tolerance problems or esophageal abnormalities. As a consequence, a range of novel BP-dosing options and formulations (intravenous) have been developed to address these varied circumstances.

A. De Sarro (✉)
Department of Clinical and Experimental Medicine and Pharmacology,
Section of Pharmacology, Faculty of Medicine and Surgery,
Policlinico Universitario "G. Martino", Messina, Italy
e-mail: desarro@unime.it

F. S. De Ponte (ed.), *Bisphosphonates and Osteonecrosis of the Jaw: A Multidisciplinary Approach*, DOI: 10.1007/978-88-470-2083-2_5,

5.1 Introduction

Osteoporosis is the most common bone disease in humans and it can affect people of all ethnic backgrounds, and especially older women and men. As such, it represents a major public health problem [1]. Osteoporosis is a disease characterized by low bone mass and microarchitectural deterioration of bone tissue, leading to enhanced bone fragility and increased susceptibility to fractures [2, 3]. Bone is a very dynamic tissue and the process of repair occurs in bone remodeling units at the surface of cortical and trabecular bone. Bone remodeling follows a time sequence that lasts about 6 months. There are five stages: (1) resting, osteoblasts become resting bone-lining cells on the newly formed bone surface; (2) *activation* of osteoclast precursors that mature into multinuclear osteoclasts under the direction of cytokines (IL-1, 2, 6, TNFα, β, TGF β) and hormones (estrogens and androgens); (3) *resorption* of bone by osteoclasts, causing a resorption cavity, a process that lasts about 3 weeks; (4) transition; and (5) *formation* of new bone that fills up the resorption cavity with new bone, a process lasting several months (Fig. 5.1) [4].

As humans age, the balance between bone formation and bone resorption is shifted in a negative direction. The number of remodeling sites across the skeleton increases under conditions of sex hormone deficiency [5]. Bone loss is the result of an imbalance in bone turnover, with bone resorption occurring at a faster rate than new bone formation. Thus, bone loss is an inevitable component of the aging process, particularly in postmenopausal women and in men with declining sex hormone levels [6]. The resulting reduction in bone mass and the accompanying damage to bone microarchitecture increase the risk of fracture. The spine (vertebral fractures), hips, and wrists (nonvertebral fractures) are the most common sites of osteoporosis-related bone fractures (i.e., fractures that are out of proportion to the level of external trauma), although osteoporosis-related fractures can occur at almost any skeletal bone site [7]. The most common form of osteoporosis, experienced by postmenopausal women, results from reduced estrogen production, which disrupts the fine balance of the bone remodeling cycle [8], and from increasing bone resorption. Osteoporosis is related to an increased risk of fractures, frequently resulting in chronic pain, disability, and death [9]. It affects approximately 26% of women and 4% of men after the age of 65 years [10, 11].

5.2 Bisphosphonates in Osteoporosis

Bisphosphonates (BPs) have been the principal anti-resorptive agents used in the therapy of osteoporosis over the last decade. Since the introduction of the first agent, alendronate, 191 million prescriptions have been written for their use [12]. Bisphosphonates work because of two key properties: (1) strong binding to bone due to a high affinity for hydroxyapatite [13, 14] and (2) the ability to inhibit osteoclast function owing to the inhibition of the enzyme farnesyl diphosphate synthase.

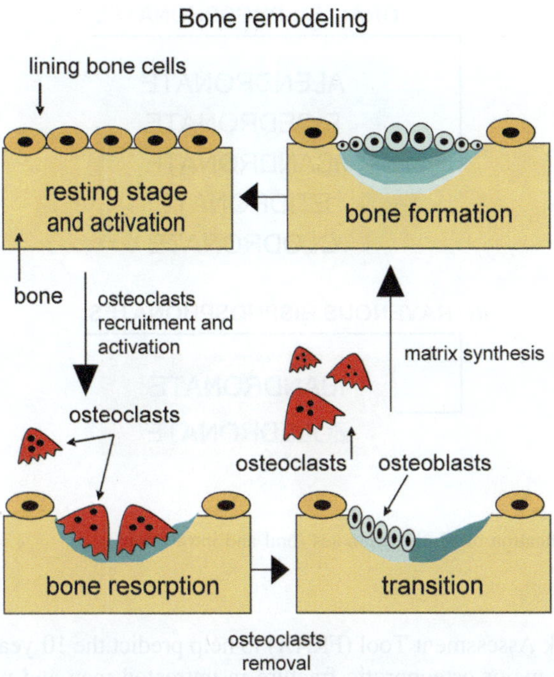

Fig. 5.1 The bone remodeling cycle. Remodeling is the replacement of old by new bone tissue that mainly occurs in the adult skeleton to maintain bone mass. This process involves the coupling of bone formation and bone resorption and consists of the following phases: *resting*, osteoblasts become resting bone-lining cells on the newly formed bone surface; *activation*, preosteoclasts are stimulated and differentiate under the influence of cytokines and growth factors into mature active osteoclasts; *resorption*, osteoclasts digest mineral matrix (old bone); *transition*, the end of resorption; and *formation*, osteoblasts synthesize new bone matrix

The Food and Drug Administration has approved the use of BPs for the treatment and/or prevention of osteoporosis. Oral alendronate (Fosamax; Merck) and oral risedronate (Actonel; Procter and Gamble Pharmaceuticals) were approved in 1995 and 2000, respectively. In 2003, oral ibandronate (Boniva; Roche Therapeutics) received approval, followed by intravenous ibandronate in 2006. Most recently, intravenous zoledronate (Reclast; Novartis) joined the market for these drugs in 2007.

Moreover, in several European countries, clodronate (a first-generation BP) has been used since 1985 for the treatment and prevention of postmenopausal osteoporosis (Fig. 5.2, Table 5.1). The diagnosis of osteoporosis relies on the quantitative assessment of bone mineral density (BMD), which correlates positively with bone strength and helps to predict future fracture risk (Fig. 5.3).

The World Health Organization (WHO) defines osteoporosis as a hip or spine BMD of $\leq$2.5 SD below the normal mean reference values for a young population, which has reached peak bone mass [15]. In addition, the WHO recently introduced

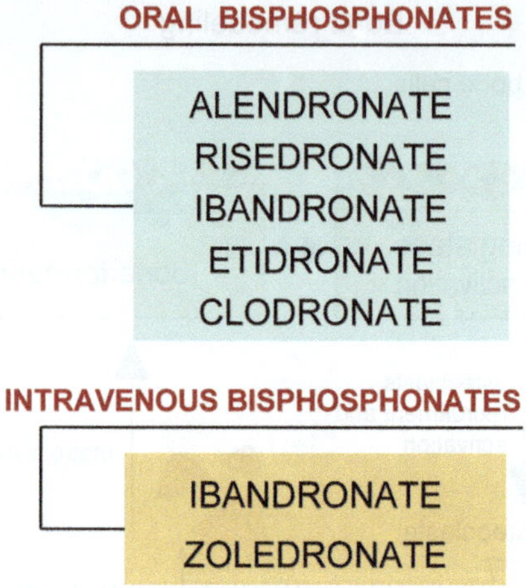

Fig. 5.2 Classification of bisphosphonates (oral and intravenous)

a Fracture Risk Assessment Tool (FRAX) to help predict the 10 year probability of a hip or other major osteoporotic fracture in untreated men and women between the ages of 40 and 90 years. The tool makes use of the femoral neck BMD as well as risk factors that are largely independent of BMD [16].

The major treatment goal for patients with osteoporosis is to prevent fractures by maintaining or increasing BMD and reducing excessive bone turnover. In fact, BPs, a mainstay among the various classes of anti-osteoporotic drugs, have been shown in numerous clinical trials to increase BMD and to reduce the risk of osteoporotic fractures [17]. Nevertheless, clinical case reports have described unusual fractures with irregular healing in cases in which an oversuppression of remodeling by BP was thought to be the cause. For example, reports of fractures of the subtrochanteric femur, pelvis, and tibia, which are uncommon in osteoporosis, focused attention on the possibility of oversuppression [18–20]. This possibiity has led some clinicians to recommend the delay of BP therapy in patients hospitalized for treatment of hip fractures, thus adding to the already difficult problem of delivering follow-up anti-fracture therapy to patients known to have osteoporosis [21, 22].

5.3 Clinical Efficacy and Safety of Bisphosphonates

Oral BPs are the current mainstay of treatment for postmenopausal osteoporosis, owing to their excellent efficacy and generally good tolerability [23–25]. However, in many cases, oral dosing options have failed to meet patient needs [22–24], enable a suitable level of adherence [26–28], or ensure optimal treatment outcomes

Table 5.1 Bisphosphonates: indication, dosage, and administration requirements

Bisphosphonate	Indications	Dosage for osteoporosis		Administration requirements (for osteoporosis)
		Prevention	Treatment	
Alendronate (Fosamax)	Prevention and treatment of osteoporosis in postmenopausal women	35 mg tablet weekly	70 mg weekly tablet or oral solution	Patient must remain upright for 30 min following dose
	Treatment to increase bone mass in men with osteporosis	5 mg tablet daily	10 mg tablet daily	
Ibandronate (Boniva)	Prevention and treatment of osteoporosis in postmenopausal women	2–5 mg tablet daily	Same as prevention dosage	*Oral (tablet)*Patient must remain upright and refrain from eating 60 min following dose
		150 mg tablet monthly		
		3 mg intravenous injection every 3 months		*Intravenous injection* 15- to 30-s bolus i.v. injection that must be administered by a health care professional
Risedronate (Actonel)	Prevention and treatment of osteoporosis in postmenopausal women	75 mg consecutive days/month	Same as prevention dosage	Patient must remain upright for 30 min following dose
	Treatment to increase bone mass in men with Osteporosis	5 mg/day		
		35 mg/weekly		
Zoledronate (Reclast)	Prevention and treatment of osteoporosis in postmenopausal women			A single 5-mg infusion once a year given intravenously over no less than 15 min in a 100-ml ready-to-infuse solution
				Administer through a separate vented infusion line and do not allow contact with any calcium- or divalent-cation-containing solutions

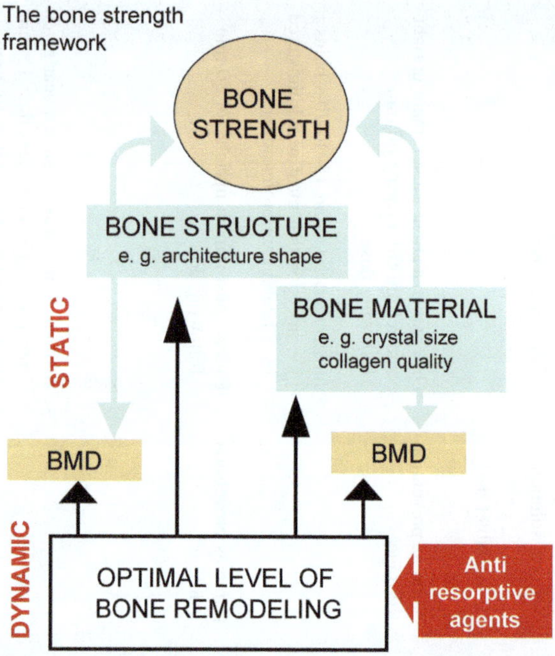

Fig. 5.3 The bone strength framework: relationship between bone mineral density and anti-resorptive agents

[29]. In fact, within 1 year of initiating treatment, more than half of all individuals taking daily or weekly BPs stop their treatment, resulting in poor effectiveness [26–29]. Moreover, for some patient groups, oral dosing is viewed as unsuitable, e.,g., in patients who cannot comply with strict dosing requirements or those who have severe upper gastrointestinal (GI) tolerance problems, or in whom oral medications may be contraindicated, as in patients with esophageal abnormalities that delay emptying.

A range of novel BP-dosing options and formulations have been developed to satisfy these varied and often complex patient circumstances. A reduction of the oral dosing frequency and thus potentially of the incidence of GI irritation may make treatment more tolerable for patients. Alternatively, the introduction of an intravenous formulation would eliminate all GI issues and might benefit those patients who cannot adhere to oral BP treatments. However, over the last decade, BPs, particularly intravenous compounds, have been associated with osteonecrosis of the jaw (ONJ) [30]. An association between intravenous BP exposure and ONJ has been hypothesized based on the following observations: (a) a positive correlation between BP potency and the risk of developing ONJ, (b) a negative correlation between BP potency and duration of BP exposure before developing ONJ, and (c) a positive correlation between the duration of BP exposure and the development of ONJ.

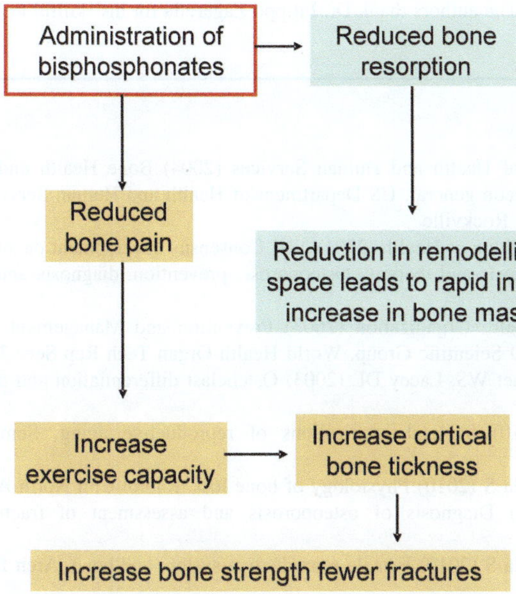

Fig. 5.4 Mechanism of action of bisphosphonates in osteoporosis

Clinical trials have shown, in some cases and at some sites, that BPs can persist in their efficacy for longer terms (7–10 years), with strong safety profiles [31, 32]. Bridging studies have assessed the efficacy of longer dosing intervals, which take advantage of the retention and recycling of BPs in the bone and have the potential to improve patient compliance and adherence during long-term treatment. These bridging trials have shown that longer dosing intervals result in equivalent benefits with respect to effect on BMD. Moreover, the availability of a once-yearly intravenous therapy (zoledronate 5 mg) may yield further improvements in compliance and outcomes in the growing population of patients with osteoporosis [33, 34].

5.4 Conclusions

- Bisphosphonates are the most widely used drugs in the treatment of osteoporosis.
- In postmenopausal women, bisphosphonates halve the osteoporotic fracture rate.
- Bisphosphonates are well tolerated, but long-term adherence to treatment is poor.
- Intermittent regimens could improve compliance.
- Some reports have suggested the potential for an increased risk of fragility fractures due to oversuppression of bone turnover with long-term bisphosphonate use (Fig. 5.4).

Acknowledgement The authors thank Dr. Filippo Zagarella for his skillful technical assistance.

References

1. US Department of Health and Human Services (2004) Bone Health and Osteoporosis: a report of the surgeon general. US Department of Health and Human Services, Office of the Surgeon General, Rockville
2. NIH National Institute of Health (2001) NIH Consensus development panel on Osteoporosis prevention, diagnosis and therapy. Osteoporosis prevention, diagnosis and therapy. JAMA 285:785–795
3. WHO World Health Organization (2003) Prevention and Management of Osteoporosis. Report of a WHO Scientific Group. World Health Organ Tech Rep Ser 921:1–164
4. Boyle WJ, Simonet WS, Lacey DL (2003) Osteoclast differentiation and activation. Nature 423:337–342
5. Freeman R (2010) Skeletal implications of reproductive aging. Semin Reprod Med 28:422–425
6. Clarke BL, Khosla S (2010) Physiology of bone loss. Radiol Clin North Am 48:483–495
7. Kanis JA (2002) Diagnosis of osteoporosis and assessment of fracture risk. Lancet 359:1929–1936
8. Clarke BL, Khosla S (2010) Female reproductive system and bone. Arch Biochem Biophys 503:118–128
9. Cummings SR, Melton LJ III (2002) Epidemiology and outcomes of osteo-porotic fractures. Lancet 359:1761–1767
10. Gaines JM, Narrett M, Parrish JM (2010) The effect of the addition of osteoporosis education to a bone health screening program for older adults. Geriatr Nurs 31:348–356
11. Rao SS, Budhwar N, Ashfaque A (2010) Bisphosphonates are the first-line agents for treating osteoporosis in men. Am Fam Physician 82:503–508
12. IMS HEALTH (2008) National prescription audit plus TM
13. Russell R (2006) Bisphosphonates: from bench to bedside. Ann N Y Acad Sci 1068:367–401
14. Nancollas GH, Tang R, Phipps RJ et al (2006) Novel insights into actions of bisphosphonates on bone: differences in interactions with hydroxyapatite. Bone 38:617–627
15. Kanis JA on behalf of the World Health Organization Scientific Group (2008) Assessment of osteoporosis at the primary health-care level. Technical Report. WHO Collaborating Centre, University of Sheffield, UK
16. Kanis JA, Johnell O, Oden A et al (2008) FRAX™ and the assessment of fracture probability in men and women from the UK. Osteoporos Int 19:385–397
17. Chapurlat RD, Delmas PD (2006) Drug insight: bisphosphonates for postmenopausal osteoporosis. Nat Clin Pract Endocrinol Metab 2:211–219
18. Goh S, Yang K, Koh J et al (2007) Subtrochanteric insufficiency fractures in patients on alendronate therapy. J Bone Joint Surg Br 89:349–353
19. Odvina CV, Zerwekh JE, Rao DS et al (2005) Severely suppressed bone turnover: a potential complication of alendronate therapy. J Clin Endocrinol Metab 90:1294–1301
20. Sellmeyer DE (2010) Atypical fractures as a potential complication of long-term bisphosphonate therapy. JAMA 304:1480–1484
21. Lenart BA, Lorich DG, Lane JM (2008) Atypical fractures of the femoral diaphysis in postmenopausal women taking alendronate. N Engl J Med 358:1304–1306
22. Giusti A, Hamdy NA, Papapoulos SE (2010) Atypical fractures of the femur and bisphosphonate therapy: A systematic review of case/case series studies. Bone 47:169–180
23. Miller PD, McClung MR, Macovei L et al (2005) Monthly oral ibandronate therapy in postmenopausal osteoporosis: 1-Year results from the MOBILE study. J Bone Miner Res 20:1315–1322

24. Sambrook PN, Rodriguez JP, Wasnich RD et al (2004) Alendronate in the prevention of osteoporosis: 7-Year follow-up. Osteoporos Int 15:483–488
25. Ste-Marie LG, Sod E, Johnson T et al (2004) Five years of treatment with risedronate and its effects on bone safety in women with postmenopausal osteoporosis. Calcif Tissue Int 75:469–476
26. Cramer JA, Amonkar MM, Hebborn A et al (2005) Compliance and persistence with bisphosphonate dosing regimens among women with postmenopausal osteoporosis. Curr Med Res Opin 21:1453–1460
27. Recker RR, Gallagher R, MacCosbe PE (2005) Effect of dosing frequency on bisphosphonate medication adherence in a large longitudinal cohort of women. Mayo Clin Proc 80:856–861
28. Penning-van Beest FJ, Goettsch WG, Erkens JA et al (2006) Determinants of persistence with bisphosphonates: A study in women with postmenopausal osteoporosis. Clin Ther 28:236–242
29. Berry SD, Misra D, Hannan MT et al (2010) Low acceptance of treatment in the elderly for the secondary prevention of osteoporotic fracture in the acute rehabilitation setting. Aging Clin Exp Res. 22:231–237
30. Durie BG, Katz M, Crowley J (2005) Osteonecrosis of the jaw and bisphosphonates. N Engl J Med 353:99–102
31. Black DM, Schwartz AV, Ensrud KE et al (2006) for the FLEX Research Group. Effects of continuing or stopping alendronate after 5 years of treatment: the Fracture Intervention Trial Long-term Extension (FLEX). A randomized trial. JAMA 296:2927–2938
32. Schnitzer T, Bone HG, Crepaldi G et al (2000) Therapeutic equivalence of alendronate 70 mg once-weekly and alendronate 10 mg daily in the treatment of osteoporosis. Aging (Milano) 12:1–12
33. Lyles KW, Colón-Emeric CS, Magaziner JS et al (2007) Zoledronic acid and clinical fractures and mortality after hip fracture. N Engl J Med 357:1799–1809
34. Reginster J-Y, Adami S, Lakatos P et al (2006) Efficacy and tolerability of once-monthly oral ibandronate in postmenopausal osteoporosis: 2 year results from the MOBILE study. Ann Rheum Dis 65:654–661

Biomorphology in BIONJ: Anatomy and Histology

6

Giuseppina Cutroneo

Abstract

The jaw is a horseshoe shaped structure with a concavity that runs dorsally. It presents an anterior and a posterior side. The jaw ramii are quadrilateral expansions that run obliquely upwards and downwards and are compressed on the lateromedial side. The mandible, which has a membranous origin, develops in the first branchial arch, where there is already a cartilaginous skeleton. A relative increase in mechanical stimulation of the jaw results in the marked neodeposition of osseous tissue that is more intensively and rapidly reabsorbed at sites not subjected to pressure. Mandibular bone is subject to normal turnover that is manifested as bone remodeling. While remodelling also involves the gingival tissue, it is unclear whether osteonecrosis of the jaw, such as occurs in patients treated with bisphosphonates, originates in the bone or in the oral mucosa. However, it has been shown that oral mucosal cells with disrupted talin function are unable to form focal adhesions and exhibit spreading defects, whereas cells with vinculin disruption can form focal adhesions but display a reduced ability to spread and an increase in cell motility.

6.1 The Jaw

The jaw bone is impar, median, and symmetric and alone constitutes the jaw bone. Its structure is horseshoe shaped, with a concavity heading dorsally and anterior and posterior sides.

G. Cutroneo (✉)
Department of Biomorphology and Biotechnologies,
University of Messina, c/o A.O.U. Policlinico Universitario "G. Martino",
Messina, Italy
e-mail: gcutroneo@unime.it

F. S. De Ponte (ed.), *Bisphosphonates and Osteonecrosis of the Jaw: A Multidisciplinary Approach*, DOI: 10.1007/978-88-470-2083-2_6,

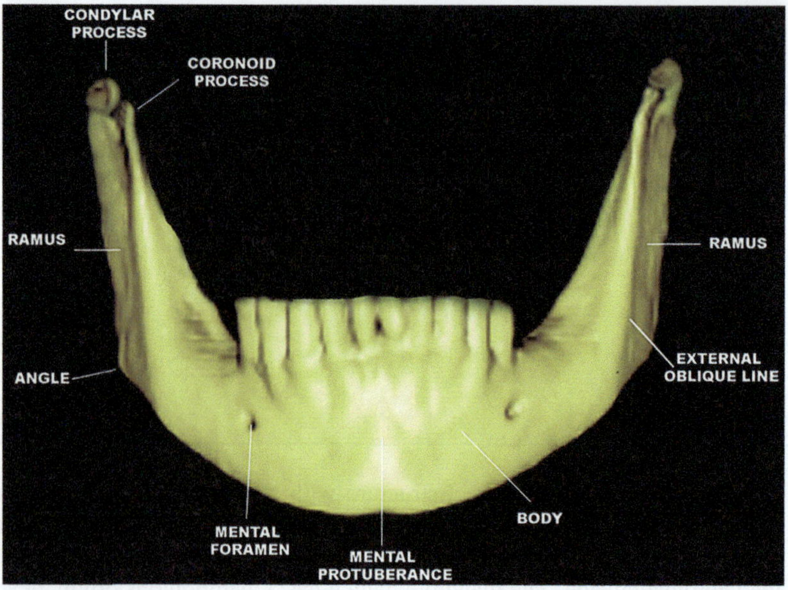

Fig. 6.1 Three-dimensional volume rendering by computed tomography scanning (in an adult). The mental protuberance and the anterior margin of the jaw ramus are seen on the anterolateral side of the jaw

The anterior or anterolateral side (Fig. 6.1) has a vertical line in its middle part, the symphysis, which is a residual of the knitting of the two halves of the bone. It terminates in its lower part with a pyramidal protrusion, the *mental protuberance*. From each side of the mental protuberance a prominent line originates, the external oblique jaw line, which forms the anterior margin of the jaw ramus. Above it, in the proximity of the second premolar, is the *mental foramen*, through which the nerve and the mental vessels pass.

The posterior or posteromedial side (Fig. 6.2), like the anterior side, is obliquely crossed by an internal oblique line, the mylohyoid line, which also links with the anterior margin of the jaw ramus and is the origin of the insertion of the mylohyoid muscle. On its medial aspect, this side presents four small eminences, the *apophysis geni*, which together form a gradual protrusion called the *mental spine*. The apophysis geni create superior insertions for the genioglossus muscles and inferior insertions for the geniohyoid muscles. From each side of the mental spine and above the mylohyoid line there is a small transverse excavation, the *sublingual fossa*, which contains the sublingual gland. Above the mylohyoid, in the proximity of the last two or three molars, a second excavation, the *submandibular fossa*, contains the submandibular gland. Parallel to the mylohyoid line is a sulcus for the mylohyoid nerve. The superior margin of the jaw is formed by sockets called *dental alveoli* (Fig. 6.3).

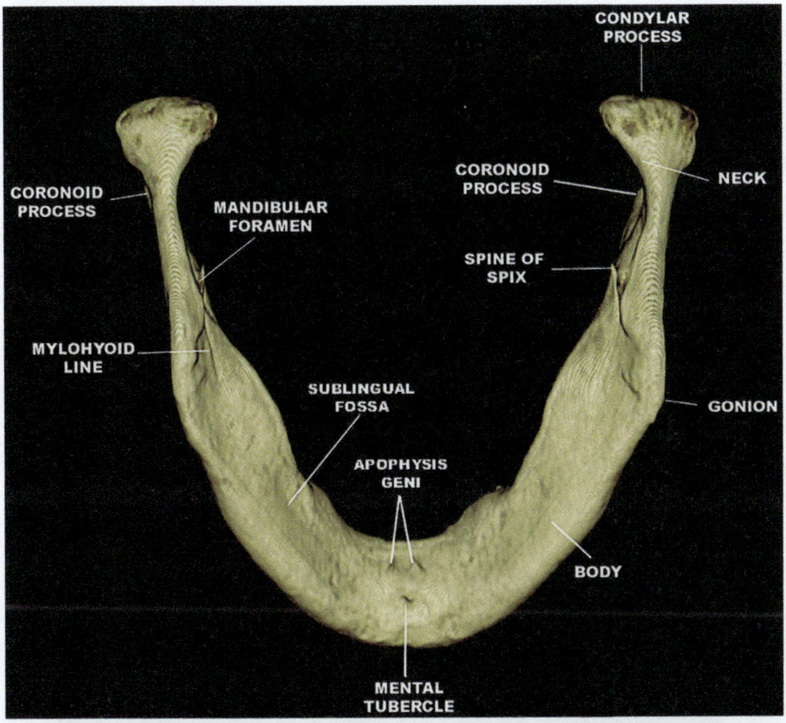

Fig. 6.2 Three-dimensional volume rendering by computed tomography scanning (in an adult). The mylohyoid line, for the mylohyoid muscle, and the apophasis geni, for the insertions of genioglossus and geniohyoid muscles are located on the posteromedial side of the jaw

The inferior margin, or bottom of the jaw, is rounded, with a very rugous oval excavation, the *digastric fossa*, on each side of the symphysis. This is the site of insertion of the anterior part of the digastric muscle.

Each half of the jaw is crossed by a long canal, the inferior alveolar canals, each of which begins on the upper internal side of the ramus in proximity to the middle part, just behind the Spix spine, heads obliquely downwards and forwards, and then continues horizontally, descending to the bottom of the dental alveolus. The canals reach the dental roots and once in the proximity of the second premolar each divides into a lateral and a medial ramus. The lateral ramus, also called the mental canal, is directed obliquely upwards; toward the outside, it reaches the external surface of the bone through the mental foramen. The medial ramus, or incisive canal, continues its course towards the symphysis and terminates below the roots of the incisors. It is placed in the spongy tissue of the bone, with various tubules originating from its upper side that ascend toward the alveolar cavity. The nerve and the alveolar vessels pass through the dental canal. The tubules constitute a passage for the collateral ramifications sent from both the nerve and the vessels to the roots of the teeth.

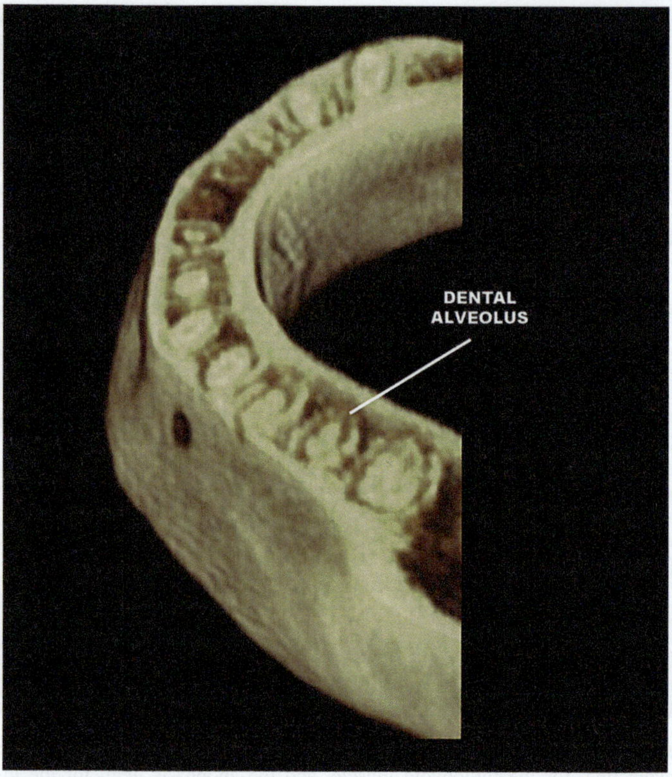

Fig. 6.3 Three-dimensional volume rendering by computed tomography scanning (in an adult). The dental alveoli are seen along the superior margin of the jaw

6.2 The Jaw Ramii

The jaw ramii are quadrilateral expansions heading obliquely upwards and downwards, forwards and backwards but compressed on the lateromedial side. They have two sides, lateral and medial. The lateral side presents robust lines aimed at the inferior insertion of the masseter muscle (Fig. 6.4). The medial side, in its central part, presents a wide orifice, the *mandibular foramen*, containing the nerve and inferior alveolar vessels. This orifice is surrounded upwards and downwards by the *Spix spine*, a triangular lamella heading vertically upwards and the site of the insertion of the sphenomandibular ligament. The inferior and posterior sides of the orifice give rise to the *mylohyoid sulcus*, heading obliquely downwards and forwards to the corpus of the bone; it is crossed by both the nerve and the mylohyoid vessels. The rugous section behind the mylohyoid sulcus, the *pterygoid tuberosity*, forms the inferior insertion of the internal pterygoid muscle (Fig. 6.5).

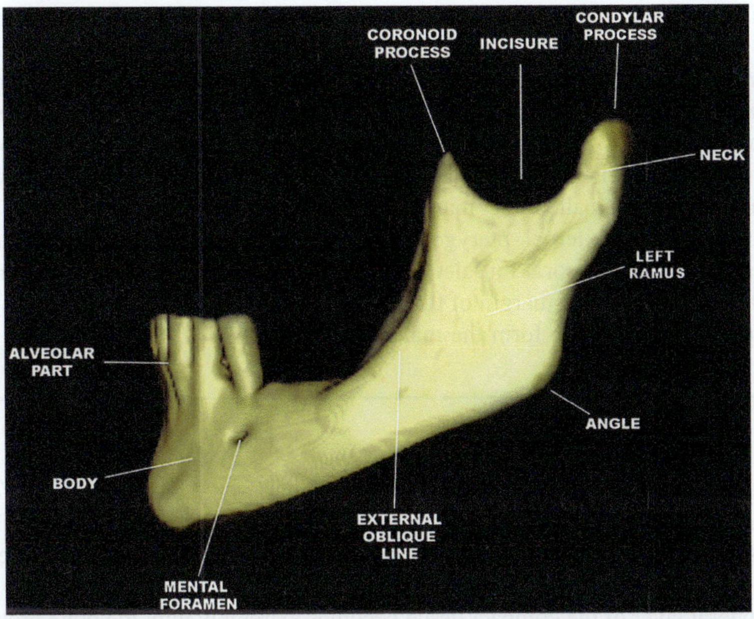

Fig. 6.4 Three-dimensional volume rendering by computed tomography scanning (in an adult). Robust lines accommodating the inferior insertion of the masseter muscle are seen along the lateral side of the jaw ramus

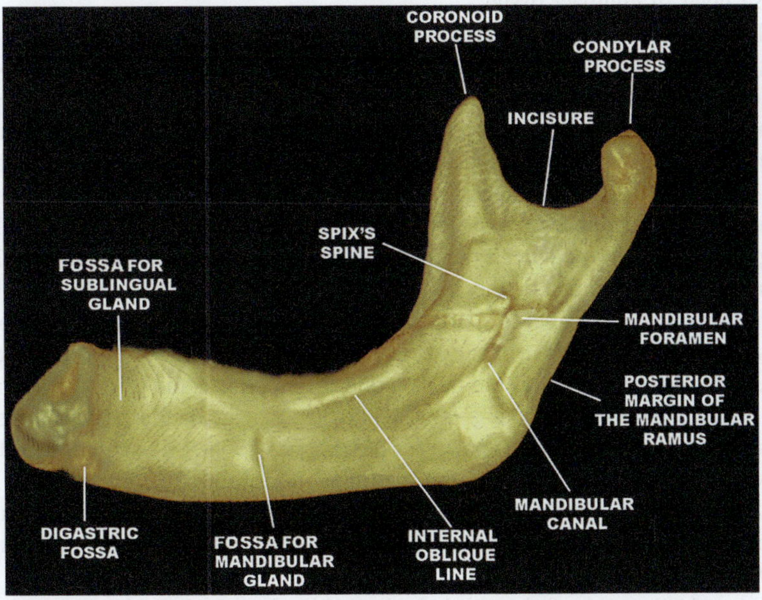

Fig. 6.5 Three-dimensional volume rendering by computed tomography scanning (in an adult). The rugosity for the inferior insertion of the internal pterygoid muscle is located on the medial side of the jaw ramus

The four margins of the jaw ramus are divided into anterior, posterior, superior, and inferior margins. The superior margin, heading backwards to forwards, is formed by two processes: anteriorly, the *coronoid process* and posteriorly the *mandibular condyle*. They are separated by a deep *sigmoid incision*. The mandibular condyle is an ellipsoid eminence, compressed on its anteroposterior side. Its long axis travels lateromedially, forwards to backwards. Below the condyle is a restricted section called the mandibular collum, the site of the fossa for the insertion of the external pterygoid muscle. The coronoid process creates the insertion for the temporal muscle. The inferior margin of the jaw ramus forms an angle with the inferior margin of the corpus and the protruding point, linking with the posterior margin to form the mandibular angle.

6.3 Histology

Histologically, the mandible has the same structure as flat bone in that it is formed by a central mass of spongy muscle tissue surrounded by a thick layer of highly resistant compact tissue (Fig. 6.6). The central tissue is very dense but near the alveolar channel it consists of spongy tissue. In the proximity of the condyle, the peripheral layer of the compact tissue becomes extremely thin: the bone protrusion is almost entirely formed by spongy tissue, whose trabeculae are mostly oriented vertically, especially in the proximity of the collum. The coronoid process, by contrast, has only a thin layer of spongy tissue that is enclosed by a very thick and dense layer of compact tissue.

The mandible, however, differs from other bones. Although it develops in the first branchial arch, where there is already cartilaginous skeleton, the mandible has a membranous origin and is formed by a center of lateral ossification, in the form of a lamina, followed by a similar center placed medially to Meckel's cartilage. The mandible's two laminae join in the lower part, creating a semicanal containing the above-mentioned cartilage, which becomes increasingly atrophied. In the semicanal, there are the nerves, alveolar vessels, and dental germs. The septal cells originate in the gaps between these germs and divide the different alveoli. In the mesenchymal thickness of the first branchial arch, which functions as a membranous skeleton, two centers of cartilage formation, anterior and posterior, are present toward the middle of the second month of fetal life. The posterior center gives rise to the first bud of the incus while the anterior is the origin of the bud of the malleus. The malleus has a long appendage that gradually pervades the arch forming Meckel's cartilage (named for the author who first illustrated it, in 1821). Towards its ventral extremity, this cartilage folds bill-like, reaching the same hooked part of the cartilage of the opposite side. With regression of the cartilage, its continuity is interrupted in the incus bud, but the modality of this regression is controversial.

Towards the end of the third fetal month, the jaw has almost reached its characteristic shape. Meckel's cartilage disappears at about the sixth month, although some trace of it will remain in the newborn. It is basically formed by two

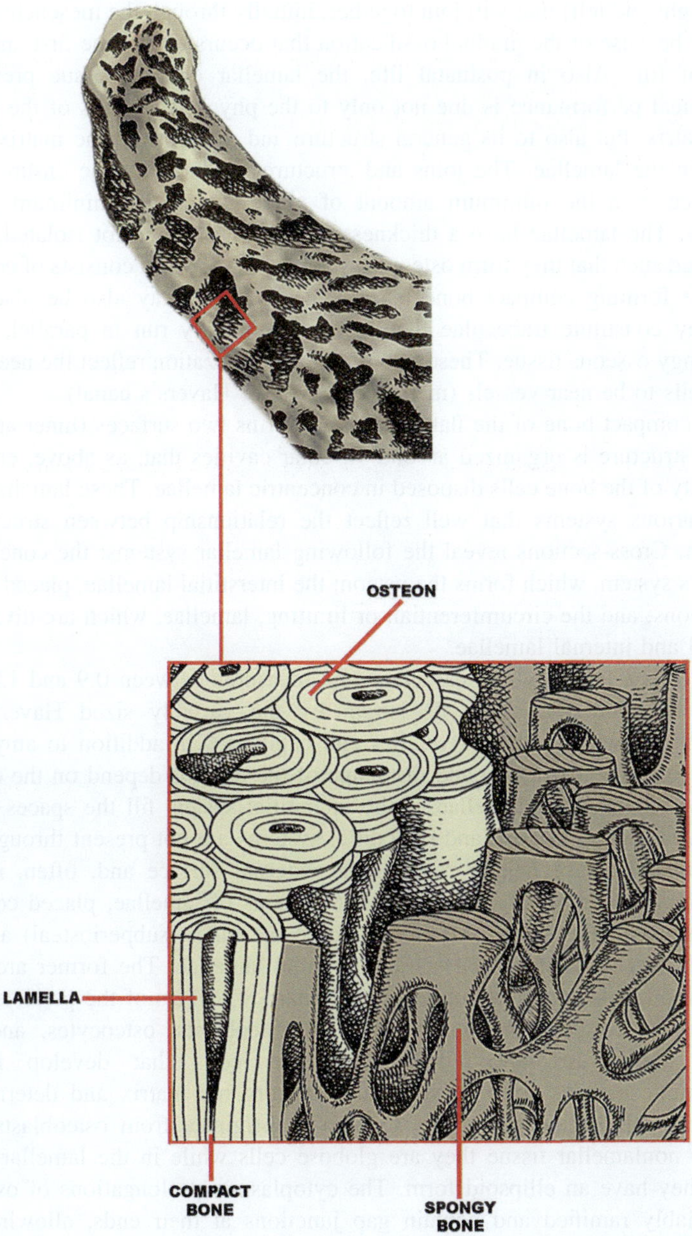

Fig. 6.6 Bone tissue of the jaw: the central tissue near the alveolar channel is made up of spongy tissue

buds (right and left) that will join together, initially through the mesenchyme, then directly because of the gradual ossification that occurs during the first and second years of life. Also in postnatal life, the lamellar osseous tissue prevails; its mechanical performance is due not only to the physical features of the extracellular matrix, but also to its general structure and therefore to the matrix's collocation in the lamellae. The joins and structures of the lamellae ensure its high resistance with the minimum amount of material and the minimum ponderal increase. The lamellae have a thickness of 4.5–11 μm, are not isolated, and are organized such that they form osteonic systems. Each osteon consists of concentric lamellae forming compact bone tissue. The lamellae may also be placed such that they constitute trabeculae that fuse to eventually run in parallel, forming the spongy osseous tissue. These two types of organization reflect the need for the bone cells to be near vessels (medullary cavity or Havers's canal).

The compact bone of the flat bone tissue forms two surfaces (inner and outer) and its structure is organized around vascular cavities that, as above, ensure the trophicity of the bone cells disposed in concentric lamellae. These lamellae join to form various systems that well reflect the relationship between structure and function. Cross-sections reveal the following lamellar systems: the concentric or Havers's system, which forms the osteon; the interstitial lamellae, placed between the osteons; and the circumferential, or limiting, lamellae, which are divided into external and internal lamellae.

The osteon has a cylindrical shape and measures between 0.9 and 1.2 mm in height. It is crossed along its length by the variably sized Haver's canal (20–110 μm) which contains venules and capillaries in addition to amyelinated nerve fibers. The regularity and the shape of the osteons depend on the extent of bone remodeling. The lamellae of the interstitial system fill the spaces between osteons. However, osteons and interstitial systems are not present throughout the entire layer because neither reaches the external surface and, often, not even the internal one. Instead, there are other systems of lamellae, placed concentric with respect to the major axis of the bone: the inner (subperiosteal) and outer (subendosteal or perimedullar) circumferential lamellae. The former are usually crossed perpendicularly and obliquely by Sharpey's fibers of the periosteum.

The cells forming the bone tissue are osteoblasts, osteocytes, and osteophages. Osteoblasts are rather voluminous cells that develop intensive osteogenetic activity since they produce the organic matrix and determine the disposition of the inorganic one. Osteocytes originate from osteoblasts; in the osseous nonlamellar tissue they are globose cells while in the lamellar osseous tissue they have an ellipsoid form. The cytoplasmic prolongations of osteocytes are variably ramified and contain gap junctions at their ends, allowing metabolic exchanges with the circulatory system. Osteophages, as their name implies, are responsible for the degradation of the osseous matrix. They are located on the bone surfaces so as to carry out resorption and often determine the formation of cavities of erosion (Howship's lacunae). Resorption and other osteophage activities are stimulated by local and systemic signals. The adhesion of osteophages to the osseous matrix is mediated by specialized, permanent structures called podosomes. Their central axis is formed by F-actin filaments surrounded by a sheath of vinculin, which, in turn, combines with talin. Therefore, podosomes can be considered as a variation of adhesion plaques and they participate in cellular anchorage to the extracellular matrix. The cytoplasm adjacent to the bone's surface contains lysosomes, which supply the enzymes needed at extracellular sites of matrix degradation. Osteophage activity that results in osteolysis occurs in two stages: demineralization and proteolysis of the matrix. Demineralization is due to the resulting decrease in pH that occurs following the release of H^+ ions (dissociation of the carbonic acid produced by carbonic anhydrase) in the area of the brush border. Proteolysis of the demineralized matrix then proceeds by lysosomal hydrolysis and metalloproteinase (collagenase) activity. The osteophage brush border is capable of actively reabsorbing the amino acids derived from proteolysis. Thus, through destruction and neo-deposition, the bones are renewed throughout life, with variable extension and rhythm in relation to age. These changes in the structure and architecture of the bones constitute remodeling. It has been amply demonstrated that a relative increase in mechanical stimulation results in the marked neo-deposition of osseous tissue that is more intensively and rapidly reabsorbed at sites not subjected to pressure. The term skeletal homeostasis indicates the life-long balance between bone structure, on the one hand, and the possible variations in mechanical stimulation on the other. Accordingly, it is important to analyze the bone tissue that, on the superior margin of the jaw, forms and envelopes the dental alveoli, which are the cavities containing the dental roots. This bone tissue, also called "alveolar bone," presents two sides: the internal side, which mediates the insertion of the fibers of the periodontal ligament, and the remaining alveolar bone. As seen in alveoli obtained because of fractures or gaps caused by dental attrition, the internal wall consists of a lamina with holes of different diameters allowing the passage of blood vessels and the insertion of the fibers of the periodontal ligament. For this reason, the internal wall of the alveolar bone is indicated as a fibrous plate or as fibrillar bone.

In radiographic images, the appearance of the internal wall is different from that of the remaining alveolar bone; it forms a small white radiodense line, the *lamina dura*. The greater compactness of the alveolar bone, without trabeculations, accounts for its radiographic features. Just like other bones, the osteophages of alveolar bones are placed along the course of the mechanical forces, thus allowing the formation of irregular trabecular bone that delimits the ample medullary spaces.

6.4 Bone Remodeling and Osteonecrosis

The high plasticity of alveolar bone enables it to adapt to the different functional necessities deriving from physiological movement or dental eruption. The latter refers not only to the emergence of the teeth, but also to the lateral movement of the tooth into the alveolus. These movements include spontaneous mesialization, which occurs in the teeth when the contiguous tooth is extracted, the lateral movements that occur in response to occlusal forces, and dental movements in response to orthodontic treatments. In general, the position of a tooth in the arcade is established when contrasting forces cancel each other out. With the teeth of the two arcades slightly distant, in the normal relaxed position of the jaw, the forces at stake are represented by the pressure exerted by the lips and by the cheeks on the external (vestibular) side and the tongue on the internal (lingual) side. However, when the teeth of the two arcades collide, the forces exerted by masticatory muscles can be divided into vertical and horizontal vectors for every contact point. The teeth will shift into the position in which the horizontal force vector is minimized. This is made possible by the minimum degree of elasticity of the periodontal ligament, but especially by the ability of the tooth to change its position in the alveolus through contemporary bone removal at sites where the ligament is compressed, together with bone deposition where the ligament is stretched, the remodeling of the fibers of the periodontal ligament, and the deposition of new cement on the radicular surface.

Once the movement is accomplished, bone absorption in the reabsorbing lacunae is typically higher than usual and is accompanied by bone deposition, thereby eliminating the irregularities of the reabsorbed surface. The first matrix to be deposited in this process contains chondroitin sulfate, followed by osteopontin, which is thought to mediate osteoblast adhesion to the surface and therefore the bone sialoproteins that precede nucleation. Fibronectin is involved only in the adhesion of osteoblasts, as are decorin and biglycan. Calcification of this very first layer essentially creates a boundary line that can be visualized through basophilic stains. The formation of new bone tracts continues above this line, followed by their transformation into lamellar bone.

The elements that permit the constant eruption of the teeth in the oral cavity and transmit to the alveolar bone the forces that cause the absorption and the reapposition of mineralized substance are fibroblasts and periodontal ligament collagen fibers. It is thought that the alveolar bone surface, in its role as the attachment site of periodontal fibers, is shorter than the surface formed by radicular cement; this is due to the small holes on the bone surface through which the vessels and nerves pass into the periodontal ligament. These holes occupy 5–10% of the useful surface of the alveolar bone and therefore constitute an alveolar wall, the *cribriform plate*. The presence of various small fibers that insert into the radicular cement and of a few large fascicles that enter the bone explain why it is more difficult for cementoblasts to reach the cement surface than for osteophages to reach the bone surface. Therefore, it can be inferred that the bone, rather than the cement, is modified through dental movements. A constant pressure exerted on the tooth provokes an increase in the number and size of the fiber fascicles, whereas a further increase of the applied strength causes bone or radicular cement remodeling; this implies a higher mobility of the tooth. In fact, the function of the periodontal ligament is to support the tooth from the inside of its alveolus; alternatively, it could be considered as the structure that enables the tooth to move

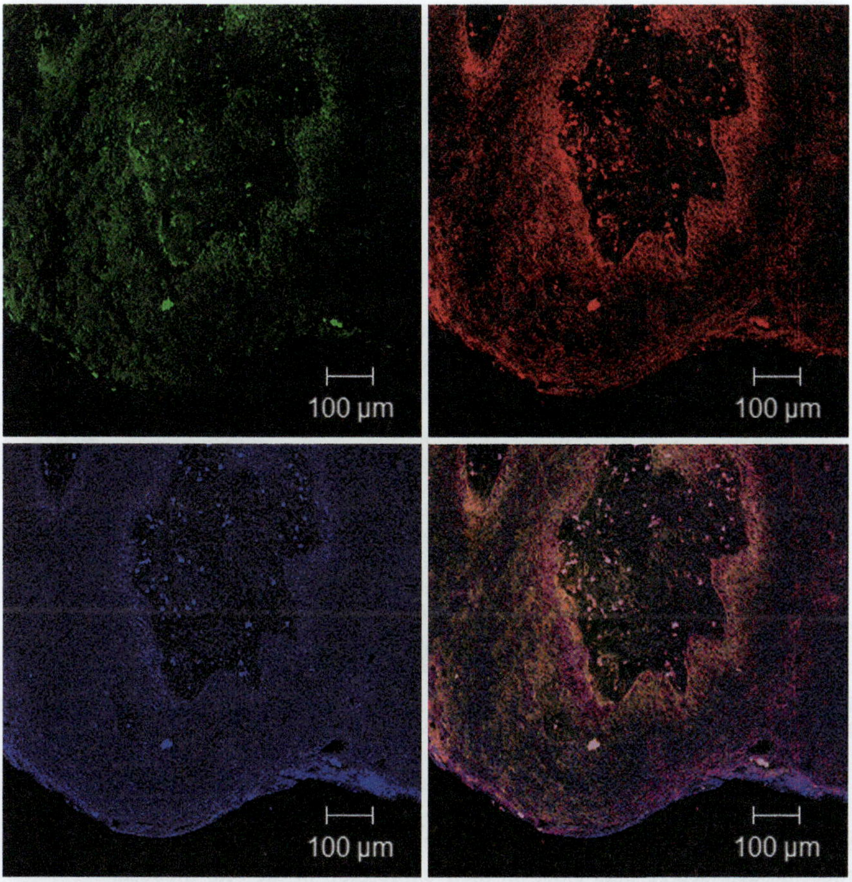

Fig. 6.7 Confocal scanning image: immunofluorescence analysis of triple localization with antibodies against talin, vinculin, and collagen in the oral mucosa of a patient treated with bisphosphonates

into the bone cavity, i.e., the alveolus of the mandibular bone, which is a rather rigid cavity. All these elements account for the integral role of the periodontal ligament within the alveolar cavities of the jaw. Indeed, the ligament can be considered as the structure that enables the jaw to maintain its normal bone structure, but it also enables normal turnover of mandibular bone and thus bone remodeling. Moreover, besides the oblique fibers, which extend from the alveolar wall towards the root of the tooth, and Sharpey's fibers, which are embedded in calcified tissues, the periodontal ligament fibres are positioned such that they keep the alveolar bone tightly adhered to the gingival tissue, in contrast to the "free fibers," which terminate in the gingival tissue. Therefore, mandibular bone remodeling is tightly associated with the gingival tissue. Although numerous

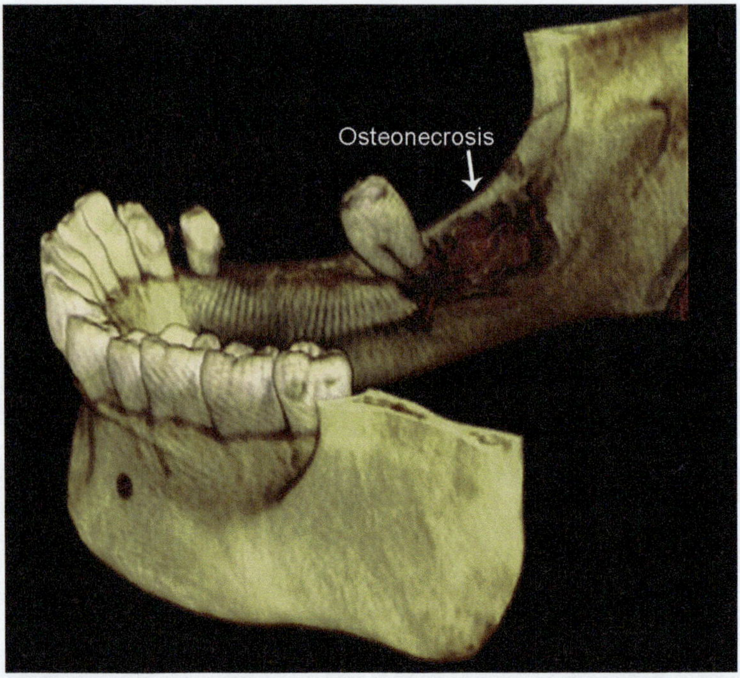

Fig. 6.8 Three-dimensional volume rendering by computed tomography scanning (in an adult). Bisphosphonate-induced osteonecrosis of the jaw

studies have been carried out on the behavior of the focal adhesion proteins in most tissues, scarce data exist on their expression in the oral mucosa.

However, it is known that oral mucosal cells with disrupted talin function are unable to form focal adhesions and exhibit spreading defects (Fig. 6.7) whereas cells in which vinculin is disrupted still form focal adhesions but their ability to spread is reduced and cell motility is increased [1, 2].

Nastro et al. [3] analyzed the human gingival mucosa of patients under treatment with bisphosphonates. They showed that all tested proteins were nearly absent or decreased in the basal lamina and oral mucosa of patients without osteonecrosis, whereas in the oral mucosa of patients with osteonecrosis of the jaw (Fig. 6.8) there was a clearly detectable staining pattern of the same proteins although at levels less than those of control samples. Therefore the authors hypothesized that osteoclast activity is suppressed in bisphosphonates-induced osteonecrosis.

This may, in turn, involve human gingival fibroblasts and human periodontal ligament cells, as both are thought to play a role in osteoclastogenesis through the expression of the receptor activator of nuclear factor kappa B ligand (RANKL) on the cell surface [4].

References

1. Priddle H, Hemmings L, Monkeley S et al (1998) Disruption of the talin gene compromises focal adhesion assembly in undifferentiated but not differentiated embryonic stem cells. J Cell Biol 142:1121–1133
2. Xu WM, Coll JL, Adamson ED (1998) Rescue of the mutant phenotype by reexpression of full-length vinculin in null F9 cells; effects on cell locomotion by domain deleted vinculin. J Cell Sci 111:1535–1544
3. Nastro Siniscalchi E, Cutroneo G, Catalfamo L et al (2010) Immunohistochemial evaluation of sarcoglycans and integrins in gingival epithelium of multiple myeloma patients with bisphosphonate-induced osteonecrosis of the jaw. Oncol Rep 24:129–134
4. Bertoldo F, Santini D, Lo Cascio V (2007) Bisphosphonates and osteomyelitis of the jaw: a pathogenic puzzle. Nat Clin Pract Oncol 4:711–721

Etiopathogenesis and Clinical Aspects of BIONJ

7

Santino Ferrara, Laura Vuolo, Annamaria Colao and Luigi Califano

Abstract

Osteonecrosis of the jaw (ONJ) was previously known as an entity mainly associated with radiation therapy to the head and neck (osteoradionecrosis of the jaw), but recent evidence of a relationship between necrotic lesions of the jaw and chronic bisphosphonates (BPs) therapy has led to a rising interest in investigating the pathogenesis of bisphosphonates-induced osteonecrosis of the jaw (BIONJ). Several studies have indicated the importance of BPs in the development of ONJ. Most published cases have described patients with advanced malignancies, particularly multiple myeloma and breast cancer, who received frequent and high doses of intravenous nitrogen-containing bisphosphonates. Advanced age, diabetes mellitus, renal insufficiency, immunosuppressant therapies such as corticosteroids, specific treatments other than BPs, alcohol consumption, cigarette smoking, among others, are considered co-morbid factors for ONJ, as the available data are conflicting and not strong enough to support these conditions as risk factors. The clinical findings in BIONJ patients include the exposure of non-vital, white-yellowish bone tissue surrounded by an inflamed and edematous mucosa in the mouth. This situation can be anticipated in patients describing a vague sensation of pain or discomfort in the affected area.

L. Califano (✉)
Stomatology and Maxillofacial Surgery,
University of Naples "Federico II", Naples, Italy
e-mail: califano@unina.it

F. S. De Ponte (ed.), *Bisphosphonates and Osteonecrosis of the Jaw: A Multidisciplinary Approach*, DOI: 10.1007/978-88-470-2083-2_7,

7.1 Etiopathogenesis of BIONJ

Osteonecrosis of the jaw (ONJ) was previously known as an entity mainly associated with radiation therapy to the head and neck (osteoradionecrosis of the jaw), but recent evidence of a relationship between necrotic lesions of the jaw and chronic bisphosphonates (BPs) therapy has led to a rising interest in investigating the pathogenesis of bisphosphonates-induced osteonecrosis of the jaw (BIONJ). BPs are powerful inhibitors of osteoclastic activity and they are widely used for the treatment of several conditions characterized by altered osteoclastic function and bone fragility, such as osteoporosis, Paget's disease, and the skeletal complications related

to cancer (osteolysis, hypercalcemeia, pathological fractures, severe pain) [1]. A definition of BIONJ, in accordance with the 2009 position paper of the American Association of Oral and Maxillofacial Surgeons states: (1) exposed necrotic bone in the maxillofacial region that persists for more than 8 weeks; (2) a history of current or previous bisphosphonates therapy; (3) no history of radiation therapy to the jaws [2].

Since its first descriptions in 2003, BIONJ has been increasingly observed in association with the use of high-dose, intravenous BP treatment and has gained considerable clinical importance. Multiple-case series and retrospective studies have focused on elucidating the etiopathogenesis of BIONJ, but many aspects are still unclear. Although several hypotheses have been advanced, the risk factors are better understood than the exact etiopatho-mechanism. Prevailing theories suggest that the most reliable risk factors are related to the effects of BPs and to findings in the jaw (Table 7.1). While there is as yet no single risk factor that alone explains the entire patho-mechanism of BIONJ, soft-tissue toxicity, an inhibition of angiogenesis, dysregulation of the immune response, and infections appear to play important roles [3–7].

7.2 Bisphosphonate-Related Risk Factors

The inhibition of osteoclastic activity is the main action of BPs, but since the activities of osteoclasts and osteoblasts are coupled, the final result is suppression of bone remodeling [8–10]. In normal bone homeostasis, osteoclastic resorption is tightly linked to osteoblastic bone deposition, and both functions are required for the repair of physiologic microdamage. In line with the *hypodynamic bone theory*, the primary mechanism for the development of ONJ in patients under BP treatment is probably the over-suppression of normal bone remodeling to an extent that local microdamage from normal mechanical loading or injury (e.g., dentoalveolar surgery or trauma) cannot be repaired, persists, and accumulates, finally leading to bone necrosis.

Several studies have indicated the importance of the *route of administration, cumulative dose, and potency* of BPs in the development of ONJ. Most published cases have described patients with advanced malignancies, particularly

Table 7.1 The main risk factors for bisphosphonate-induced osteonecrosis of the jaw

Bisphosphonates-related risk factors
Potency
Treatment duration
Anti-angiogenic properties
Soft-tissue toxicity
Local risk factors
Dentoalveolar surgery or trauma
Local anatomic structure: exostosis or prominences (tori)
Concomitant endodontitis, periodontitis, infections

multiple myeloma and breast cancer, who received frequent and high doses of intravenous nitrogen-containing bisphosphonates (N-BPs). Of these, zoledronate and pamidronate are associated with a much greater risk than non-N-BPs. Estimates of the incidence of BIONJ in patients receiving intravenous BPs range from 0.8 to 12%, with a clearly lower incidence in patients taking oral BPs to treat non-malignant bone diseases such as osteoporosis, rheumatoid arthritis, and Paget's disease.

The most striking difference between these oral and intravenous administration is the bioavailability of the drug. Oral bioavailability is around 1% due to higher ionization at physiologic pH when the drug is adsorbed by the intestinal mucosa. The greater bioavailability, high cumulative doses, and high potency of intravenous BPs explain the significantly higher incidence of ONJ in this group [1–3].

Based on published data, it has become clear that longer duration of BP treatment and a higher cumulative dose of these drugs are associated with the development of ONJ. Many studies revealed that these patients had received greater doses of BPs and for a longer period than was the case in non-ONJ patients. A recent study conducted on 3,994 patients showed that cases of ONJ were associated with significantly longer median duration of pamidronate (1.68 vs. 0.59 years in breast cancer and 1.55 vs. 0.30 years in multiple myeloma) and zoledronic acid (2.04 vs. 0.73 years in breast cancer and 1.85 vs. 0.67 years in myeloma) treatment [11]. Furthermore, the onset of jawbone necrosis is likely related not only to the cumulative dose of BPs but also to their potency and type. Both factors define the degree of bone remodeling inhibition, since in initial reports the risk of developing ONJ was greater with zoledronic acid than with other BPs [12, 13].

In concert with the direct effects of BPs on bone cells, another potential mechanism to explain BIONJ is based on the drugs' anti-angiogenic properties, given that osteoclasts differentiate from hematopoietic precursor cells. Some authors have suggested that BPs promote avascular necrosis of the jaw by inducing obliteration of the regional blood vessels [14–16]. BPs, particularly N-BPs, are thought to exert several adverse effects on the local blood supply. The mechanism of these effects may be attributable to a complex interaction of BPs with growth hormone (GH) and insulin-like growth factor I (IGF-I), both of which are involved in regulating the circulation in bones. BPs were shown to inhibit endothelial cell function in vitro and in vivo and to significantly decrease circulating levels of vascular endothelial growth factor (VEGF), a potent angiogenic factor, resulting in reduced capillary-tube formation [17, 18]. Since these properties were not recognized during the trial stages of these drugs, it can be hypothesized that the ischemic effects are cumulative over time. The vascular supply to the mandible is inherently restricted whereas the maxilla is well supplied by the vasculature.

Moreover, some studies suggest that BPs also exert effects on soft tissues, with direct toxicity to the oral mucosa, thus contributing to mucosal fenestration and bone exposure [5].

7.2.1 Local Risk Factors

Localization of the damage to the jaw can be explained by the constant stress of strong occlusal masticatory forces. The heightened daily bone remodeling requirements lead to higher concentrations of BPs being taken up in the jaws. That is, given that the bones of the jaw are sites of elevated bone turnover, BP levels within the maxilla and mandible would be selectively elevated [2]. Furthermore, the necrosis is more common in areas where a thin mucosa covers a bony exostosis or bony prominences such as lingual, mylohyoid, and palatal tori [14, 19]. Most (50–80%) cases of BIONJ are preceded by dentoalveolar surgery or dental trauma [11, 20–23]. Dental procedures, such as extractions or implants, are recognized as precipitating events since they increase the demand for osseous repair that exceeds the capacity of the hypodynamic bone, resulting in localized bone necrosis. Recent data indicated that the risk of developing ONJ was 53 times higher in patients with previous dental extraction than in patients who had not had a dental extraction during BPs treatment [24, 25]. Physiologically, no complications occur in the healing of a wound in the oral cavity, but when the mandible or maxilla is injured by a pathological process or high radiation doses, the reduced healing potential could increase the risk of necrosis and osteomyelitis at these sites [2].

Moreover, the mandible and maxilla are more frequently the site of infection than all other bones in the body. The jaw is separated from the oral cavity, an area vulnerable to trauma and microbiologically diverse, by a fragile barrier consisting of a thin mucosa and periosteum. Also, profound caries, endodontitis, and periodontitis further contribute to the onset of infections involving the bones of the jaw.

Recently, a novel etiopathogenetic mechanism linking BPs, local infections, and local pH was proposed. Both infections and dentoalveolar surgery have the potential to lower the pH (acidosis) of the oral cavity and associated structures.

Physiologically, BPs bind to the bone at neutral pH and dissociate from hydroxyapatite in an acidic milieu. Thus, the consequences of a decrease in pH are not only direct cytotoxic effects on different cells, but also a local increase in active BPs. A recent study conducted by Otto et al. investigated the effects of the N-BPs zoledronate, ibandronate, and the non-N-BP clodronate at different concentrations and at different pH values (7.4, 7.0, 6.7, and 6.3) on mesenchymal stem cells in vitro. The results showed that high doses of N-BPs and a local acidic milieu, such as are frequently present in infections of the jaw, caused a significant decrease in cell survival and activity. Both zoledronate and ibandronate exhibited dose- and pH-dependent cellular toxicity, whereas the response of cells exposed to equimolar concentrations of clodronate was comparable to that in the BP-free controls [3]. These results may be explained by the protonated activation of N-BPs at low pH [26–28].

7.2.2 Predisposing Factors

Advanced age, diabetes mellitus, renal insufficiency, immunosuppressant therapies such as corticosteroids, specific treatments other than BPs, alcohol consumption, cigarette smoking, among others, are considered co-morbid factors for ONJ, as the available data are conflicting and not strong enough to support these conditions as risk factors. Some studies have suggested that neither treatments for breast cancer, such as anthracyclines, tamoxifen, taxanes, trastuzumab, and aromatase inhibitors, nor multiple myeloma treatments, such as anthracyclines, melphalan, and thalidomide, nor patient age, renal insufficiency, alcohol use, and smoking were significantly associated with a greater risk for ONJ [24]. In contrast, others showed a correlation between cyclophosphamide or erythropoietin use in multiple myeloma patients, advanced age, and renal dialysis and the development of ONJ. Moreover, according to recent studies, patients under treatment with the anti-angiogenic drug bevacizumab for metastatic cancers have a greater risk of developing ONJ, while the anti-angiogenic drug sunitinib has been linked with ONJ progression [29–32]. The role of glucocorticoids in the development of necrosis of the jaw remains unclear, but it is well known that the long-term use of systemic steroids promotes aseptic necrosis of the bones, particularly of the femoral heads. However, based on published data, it is probable that high cumulative doses of glucocorticoids are a triggering factor for ONJ [24, 33–35]. Finally, because BP users develop bone necrosis only rarely, individual genetic variations in drug metabolism may influence susceptibility or resistance to BIONJ [2]. A study conducted among multiple myeloma patients treated with intravenous BPs demonstrated an association between a single-nucleotide polymorphism in the cytochrome P450-2C gene (CYP2C8) and an increased risk of BIONJ [36].

Thus, summarizing, BIONJ encompasses a wide range of etiologic factors and may result from one or more of them. It is now well established that intravenous BPs and dentoalveolar procedures are the main risk factors for BIONJ.

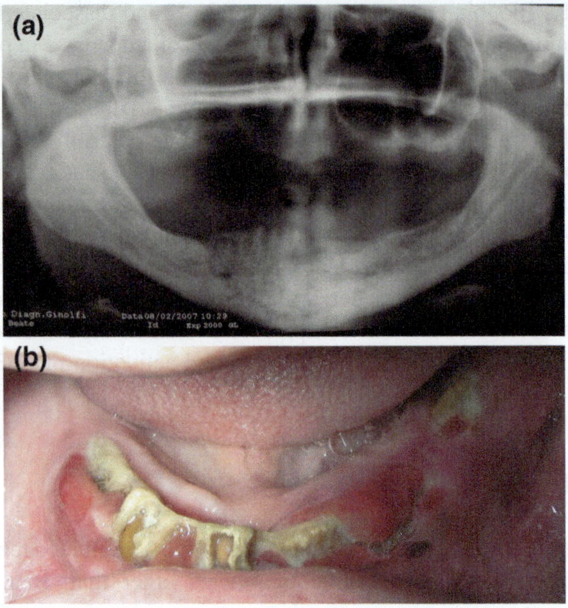

Fig. 7.1 **a** Osteonecrosis of the mandible, **b** in a completely edentulous patient

7.3 Clinical Aspects of BIONJ

The clinical findings in BIONJ patients include the exposure of non-vital, white-yellowish bone tissue surrounded by an inflamed and edematous mucosa in the mouth. This situation can be anticipated in patients describing a vague sensation of pain or discomfort in the affected area.

As previously described, osteonecrosis generally develops after procedures that cause trauma to the jaw (e.g., dental extractions). Episodes of spontaneous onset have been reported and documented and are more likely to occur close to palatal and mandibular tori and in partially or completely edentulous patients (Fig. 7.1). The early signs and symptoms of BIONJ are the same as in any odontogenous infection (halitosis, pain, edema and ulceration of the mucosa, dental mobility). In an advanced stage of the disease, there may be inflammatory and infectious foci (suppurative osteomyelitis), pathological fractures, skin fistulas, as well as oral and nasal antral fistulas, all of which contribute to worsen the symptomatology. Patients at risk for or with established BIONJ may also present with other common clinical conditions, including alveolar osteitis, sinusitis, gingivitis/periodontitis, caries, periapical pathology, and temporomandibular joint disorders [1]. Diagnosis is based on clinical findings rather than on histological or radiographic evidence. Radiographically, the condition has a normal appearance or it may resemble

Table 7.2 Staging of BIONJ (from [37])

Stage 0	Subclinical condition, microscopically characterized by initial hypocellularity and apoptosis of osteoclasts, reduction of endosteal osteoblasts, and reduction of osteoid tissue synthesis
Stage 1a	Painless bone exposure <1 cm
Stage 1b	Painless bone exposure >1 cm
Stage 2a	Single exposed area <2 cm associated with pain and/or clinical signs of infection
Stage 2b	Single exposed area >2 cm associated with pain and/or clinical signs of infection
Stage 3a	Multiple areas of bone exposure without clinical signs of osteolysis, oral cutaneous fistulas, or pathological fractures
Stage 3b	Area of bone exposure >3 cm or areas with clinical signs of osteolysis or oral cutaneous fistula, or pathological fracture

bacterial osteomyelitis or osteoradionecrosis. The clinical appearance and history are sufficient to distinguish ONJ from other delayed bone and wound-healing pathologies [37].

The position paper of the American Association of Oral and Maxillofacial Surgeons (AAOMS) on BIONJ, published in 2009, identified five different categories for BIONJ staging [1]:

"At risk": No evidence of necrotic bone in patients treated with oral or intravenous bisphosphonates

Stage 0: No clinical evidence of necrotic bone, but non-specific clinical findings and symptoms

Stage 1: Exposed and necrotic bone in patients who are asymptomatic and have no evidence of infection

Stage 2: Exposed and necrotic bone in patients with pain and clinical evidence of infection

Stage 3: Exposed and necrotic bone in patients with pain, infection, and one or more of the following: necrotic-bone exposure extending beyond the region of alveolar bone (i.e., inferior border and ramus in the mandible, maxillary sinus and zygoma in the maxilla) resulting in pathological fracture, extra-oral fistula, oral antral/oral nasal communication, and/or osteolysis extending to the inferior border of the mandible or sinus floor [1]

The BP-induced exposure of bone is also scored by clinical severity. Marx proposed a clinical staging of bone exposure in ONJ (Table 7.2) in which the exposed bone is necrotic but not sore, is classified as stage 1a if the exposed area measures <1 cm (Fig. 7.1) and stage 1b if >1 cm (Fig. 7.2). Single exposed areas, accompanied by pain and/or clinical infection, measuring >2 cm are classified

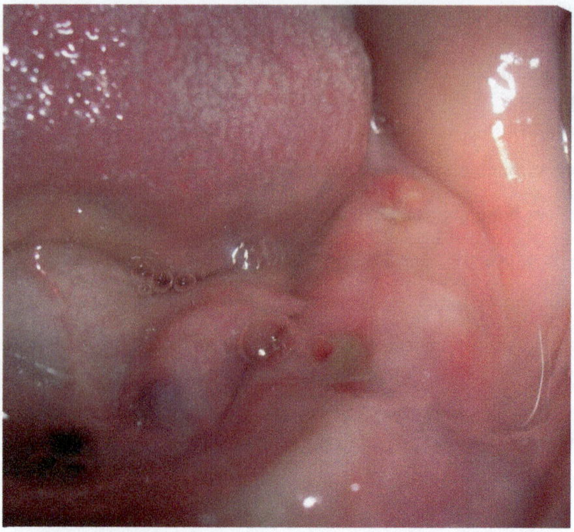

Fig. 7.2 Stage 1a: exposed bone area <1 cm

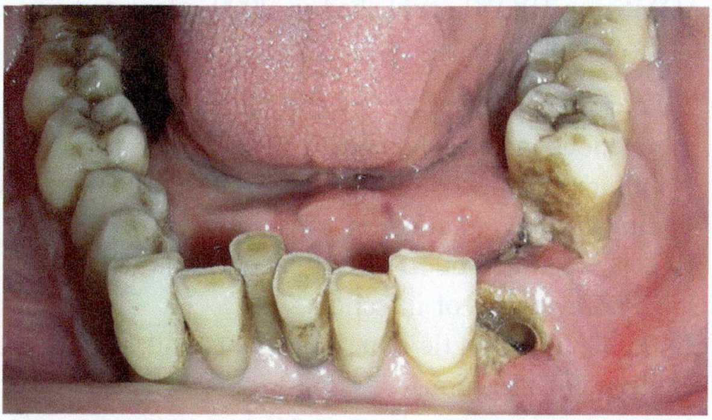

Fig. 7.3 Stage 1b: exposed bone area >1 cm

as stage 2a (Fig. 7.3) and if >2 cm then stage 2b (Fig. 7.4). Multiple areas of bone exposure without significant osteolysis, orocutaneous fistulas, or pathological fractures are classified as stage 3a (Fig. 7.5); lesions with an area of bone exposure >3 cm, or all lesions associated with significant osteolysis (Fig. 7.6) or orocutaneous fistulas (Fig. 7.7) or pathological fractures (Fig. 7.8) are classified as stage 3b [37]. Once the bone is exposed, it remains permanently exposed with no possibility of spontaneous resolution, even if the BPs are suspended (Fig. 7.9).

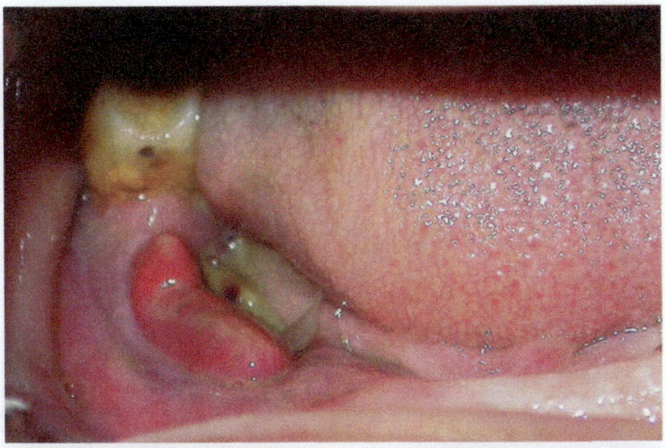

Fig. 7.4 Stage 2a: exposed bone area <2 cm

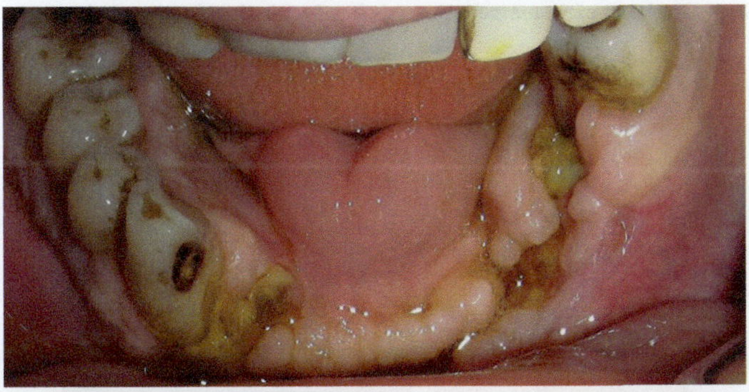

Fig. 7.5 Stage 2b: bone exposure area >2 cm

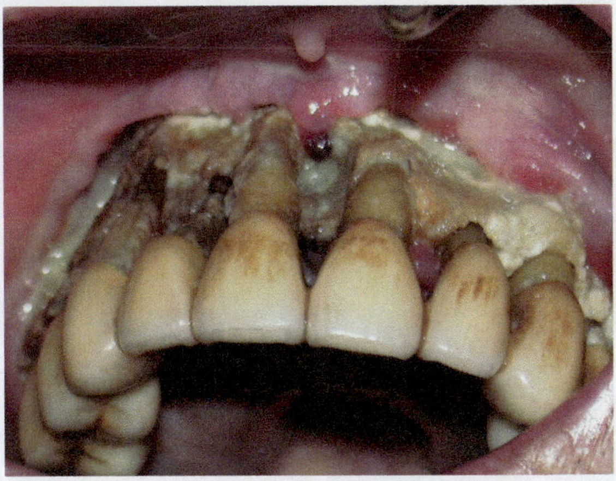

Fig. 7.6 Stage 3a: multiple areas of bone exposure without significant osteolysis, oral cutaneous fistulas, or pathological fractures

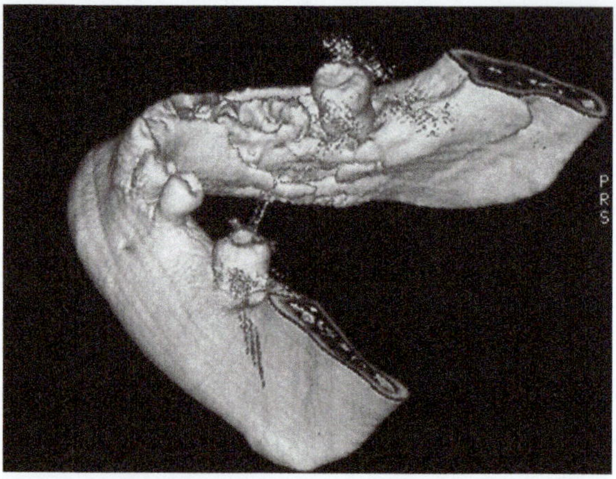

Fig. 7.7 Stage 3b: bone exposure >3 cm, associated with significant osteolysis

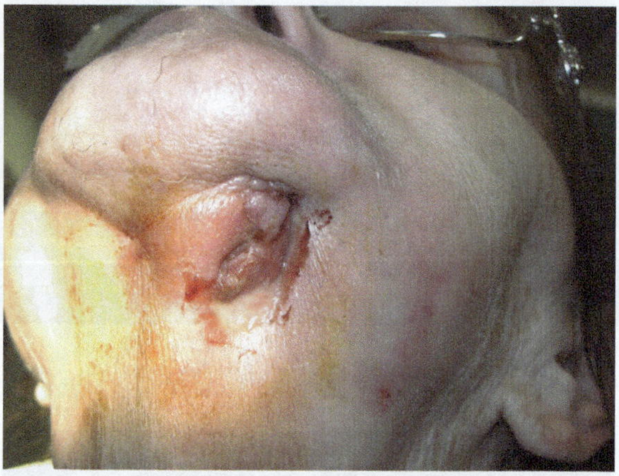

Fig. 7.8 Stage 3b: bone exposure and oral cutaneous fistulas

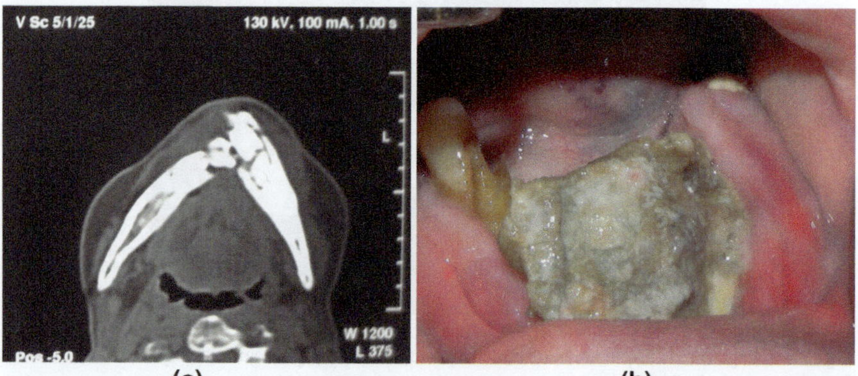

Fig. 7.9 **a** Pathological fractures associated, **b** with stage 3b bone exposure

The treatment objectives for patients with an established diagnosis of BIONJ are to eliminate pain, control infection of the soft and hard tissues, and minimize the progression or occurrence of bone necrosis.

References

1. Ruggiero SL (2010) Bisphosphonate-related osteonecrosis of the jaw: an overview. Ann NY Acad Sci Sep 28 doi:10.1111/j.1749-6632.2010.05768.x
2. Ruggiero SL, Dodson TB, Assael LA et al (2009) American association of oral and maxillofacial surgeons position paper on bisphosphonate-related osteonecrosis of the jaws: update. J Oral Maxillofac Surg 67(Suppl 5):2–12
3. Otto S, Pautke C, Opelz C et al (2010) Osteonecrosis of the jaw: effect of bisphosphonate type, local concentration, and acidic milieu on the pathomechanism. J Oral Maxillofac Surg 68(11):2837–2845
4. Reid IR, Bolland MJ, Grey AB (2007) Is bisphosphonate-associated osteonecrosis of the jaw caused by soft tissue toxicity? Bone 41:318
5. Landesberg R, Cozin M, Cremers S et al (2008) Inhibition of oral mucosal cell wound healing by bisphosphonates. J Oral Maxillofac Surg 66:839–847
6. Cetinkaya BO, Keles GC, Ayas B et al (2008) Effects of risedronate on alveolar bone loss and angiogenesis: a stereologic study in rats. J Periodontol 79:1950
7. Deckers MM, Van Beek ER, Van Der Pluijm G et al (2002) Dissociation of angiogenesis and osteoclastogenesis during endochondral bone formation in neonatal mice. J Bone Miner Res 17:998
8. Fleisch H (2002) The role of bisphosphonates in breast cancer: development of bisphosphonates. Breast Cancer Res 4(1):30–34
9. Russell RG (2007) Bisphosphonates: mode of action and pharmacology. Pediatrics 119(Suppl 2): S150–S162
10. Almazrooa SA, Woo SB (2009) Bisphosphonate and nonbisphosphonate-associated osteonecrosis of the jaw: a review. J Am Dent Assoc 140(7):864–875
11. Weinstein RS, Roberson PK, Manolagas SC (2009) Giant osteoclast formation and long-term oral bisphosphonate therapy. N Engl J Med 360:53
12. Hoff AO, Toth B, Hu M et al (2010) Epidemiology and risk factors for osteonecrosis of the jaw in cancer patients. Ann NY Acad Sci doi:10.1111/j.1749-6632.2010.05771.x
13. Nancollas GH, Tang R, Phipps RJ et al (2006) Novel insights into actions of bisphosphonates on bone: differences in interactions with hydroxyapatite. Bone 38:617
14. Marx RE, Sawatari Y, Fortin M et al (2005) Bisphosphonate induced exposed bone (osteonecrosis/osteopetrosis) of the jaws: risk factors, recognition, prevention, and treatment. J Oral Maxillofac Surg 63:1567–1575
15. Ruggiero SL, Mehrotra B, Rosenberg TJ et al (2004) Osteonecrosis of the jaws associated with the use of bisphosphonates: a review of 63 cases. J Oral Maxillofac Surg 62:527–534
16. Koch FP, Merkel C, Ziebart T et al (2010) Influence of bisphosphonates on the osteoblast RANKL and OPG gene expression in vitro. Clin Oral Invest doi:10.1007/s00784-010-0477-8
17. Santini D, Vincenzi B, Avvisati G (2002) Pamidronate induces modifications of circulating angiogenic factors in cancer patients. Clin Cancer Res 8:1080–1084
18. Wood J, Bonjean K, Ruetz S (2002) Novel antiangiogenic effects of the bisphosphonate compound zolendronic acid. J Pharmacol Exp Ther 302:1055–1061
19. Estilo CL, Van Posnak CH, Williams T et al (2004) Osteonecrosis of the maxilla and mandible in patients treated with bisphosphonates: a retrospective study. J Clin Oncol Proc Am Soc Clin Oncol 22:8088

20. Khosla S, Burr D, Cauley J et al (2007) Bisphosphonate-associated osteonecrosis of the jaw: report of a task force of the American Society for Bone and Mineral Research. J Bone Miner Res 22:1479
21. Abu-Id MH, Warnke PH, Gottschalk J et al (2008) "Bis-phossy jaws"—high and low risk factors for bisphosphonate-induced osteonecrosis of the jaw. J Craniomaxillofac Surg 36:95
22. Kyrgidis A, Vahtsevanos K, Koloutsos G et al (2008) Bisphosphonaterelated osteonecrosis of the jaws: a case-control study of risk factors in breast cancer patients. J Clin Oncol 26:4634
23. Lo JC, O'Ryan FS, Gordon NP et al (2010) Predicting risk of osteonecrosis of the jaw with oral Bisphosphonate Exposure (PROBE) Investigators. Prevalence of osteonecrosis of the jaw in patients with oral bisphosphonate exposure. J Oral Maxillofac Surg 68:243
24. Hoff AO, Toth BB, Altundag K et al (2008) Frequency and risk factors associated with osteonecrosis of the jaw in cancer patients treated with intravenous bisphosphonates. J Bone Miner Res 23:826
25. Hess LM, Jeter JM, Benham-Hutchins M et al (2008) Factors associated with osteonecrosis of the jaw among bisphosphonate users. Am J Med 121:475
26. Otto S, Hafner S, Mast G et al (2010) Bisphosphonate-related osteonecrosis of the jaw: is pH the missing part in the pathogenesis puzzle? J Oral Maxillofac Surg 68:1158
27. Russell RG, Watts NB, Ebetino FH et al (2008) Mechanisms of action of bisphosphonates: similarities and differences and their potential influence on clinical efficacy. Osteoporos Int 19:733
28. Leu CT, Luegmayr E, Freedman LP et al (2006) Relative binding affinities of bisphosphonates for human bone and relationship to antiresorptive efficacy. Bone 38:628
29. Greuter S, Schmid F, Ruhstaller T et al (2008) Bevacizumab-associated osteonecrosis of the jaw. Ann Oncol 19(12):2091–2092
30. Estilo CL, Fornier M, Farooki A et al (2008) Osteonecrosis of the jaw related to bevacizumab. J Clin Oncol 26(24):4037–4038
31. McArthur HL, Estilo C, Huryn J et al (2008) Osteonecrosis of the jaw (ONJ) among intravenous (IV) bisphosphonate- and/or bevacizumab-treated patients (pts) at Memorial Sloan-Kettering Cancer Center (MSKCC). J Clin Oncol 26(155):9588
32. Brunello A, Saia G, Bedogni A et al (2009) Worsening of osteonecrosis of the jaw during treatment with sunitinib in a patient with metastatic renal cell carcinoma. Bone 44(1):173–175
33. Jadu F, Lee L, Pharoah M et al (2007) A retrospective study assessing the incidence, risk factors and comorbidities of pamidronate-related necrosis of the jaws in multiple myeloma patients. Ann Oncol 18:2015–2019
34. Gebhard KL, Maibach HI (2001) Relationship between systemic corticosteroids and osteonecrosis. Am J Clin Dermatol 2(6):377–388
35. Assouline-Dayan Y, Chang C, Greenspan A et al (2002) Pathogenesis and natural history of osteonecrosis. Semin Arthritis Rheum 32(2):94–124
36. Sarasquete M (2008) BRONJ is associated with polymorphisms of the cytochrome P450 CYP2C8 in multiple myeloma: a genome-wide single nucleotide analysis. Blood 111:2709
37. Marx RE (2009) L'osteonecrosi dei Mascellari da bisfosfonati. Quintessence, Milan

Instrumental Diagnosis

8

Silvio Mazziotti, Achille Mileto, Michele Gaeta, Giorgio Ascenti, Ignazio Salamone, Carmela Visalli and Alfredo Blandino

Abstract

In the diagnosis of osteonecrosis of the jaw (ONJ), imaging may have a role in determining the extent of the disease, diagnosing early stages of osteonecrosis, identifying a potential association between metastasis to the jaw and ONJ lesions, excluding other diseases or complications of the jaws, such as fractures, and evaluating the jaw before surgical orofacial procedures. Since the appearance of ONJ at imaging is variable and very often nonspecific, imaging findings should always be related to the clinical context. The panoramic radiograph is the most often used imaging technique in cases of ONJ, whereas CT and MRI are adequate in evaluating bone involvement, in addition to offering the advantage that destructive processes can be seen at high resolution. Functional imaging, especially bone scintigraphy, provides a tool for the detection of early stages of ONJ.

8.1 Introduction

The diagnosis of osteonecrosis of the jaw (ONJ) is primarily clinical and is generally established at a late stage of the disease, since patients usually come to the attention of the clinician when osteonecrosis is already symptomatic [1, 2].

Imaging may have a role in determining the extent of the disease, diagnosing early stages of osteonecrosis, identifying a potential association between metastasis to the jaw and ONJ lesions, excluding other diseases or complications of the

A. Blandino (✉)
Department of Radiological Sciences,
University of Messina, Policlinico "G.Martino",
Messina, Italy
e-mail: ablandino@unime.it

F. S. De Ponte (ed.), *Bisphosphonates and Osteonecrosis of the Jaw: A Multidisciplinary Approach*, DOI: 10.1007/978-88-470-2083-2_8,

jaws, such as fractures, and evaluating the jaw before surgical orofacial procedures [3, 4]. It is important to add that the imaging appearance of ONJ is variable and very often nonspecific, and should always be related to the clinical context [1–3]. Nevertheless, different imaging modalities have been proposed for the detection of ONJ [2–4].

The panoramic radiograph is the most often used imaging technique in cases of ONJ [5]. Computed tomography (CT) and magnetic resonance imaging (MRI) are also appropriate for evaluating bone involvement and offer the advantage that destructive processes can be seen at high resolution. Moreover, three-dimensional images can be generated if necessary.

Besides CT and MRI, functional imaging (bone scintigraphy) has been proposed for the detection of early stages of ONJ. However, bone scintigraphy is limited due to its low spatial resolution, difficulty in differentiating between inflammatory and malignant processes, and the fact that metric analyses are not possible with this technique [6].

8.2 Panoramic Radiograph and CT

Panoramic radiographs are typically employed as the first line in routine radiologic evaluation, as the observed abnormalities may appear more extensive than the clinical lesions [3, 4]. The appearance of ONJ at panoramic radiograph is variable; indeed, bone may appear normal when the lesions are <1 cm [3–5]. Although panoramic radiography provides sufficient information for primary diagnosis and monitoring of the disease process, it is relatively insensitive in demonstrating the extent of the lesions or complications such as fractures [3–5].

Some studies have concluded that panoramic radiography is less sensitive than CT [4, 5, 7]. Others have stated that panoramic radiography is better than CT in providing additional information about the extent of symptomatic lesions and lesions without exposed bone [4, 5, 7, 8]. Globally, panoramic radiographic and CT findings present as ill-defined areas of lucency or low attenuation. There may be a thickened and disorganized medullary trabeculation, permeative appearance, cortical disruption, increased thickness of the lamina dura and mandibular canal margins, bone sequestrum, periosteal bone formation, or osteosclerosis. The bone changes may be mixed, predominantly lytic, or predominantly sclerotic [4, 5, 7–9].

CT is the best modality to provide information about cortical and trabecular bone as it allows estimations of the extent of the necrotic process and distinguishes ONJ from malignant diseases such as plasmocytoma or bone metastases [5, 7–9]. Focal medullary sclerosis with disorganized microtrabeculae and poor corticomedullary differentiation in the suspected necrotic site has been described as a finding associated with early symptoms of tooth loosening. Persistent alveolar sockets related to delayed socket healing, especially after teeth extractions, are a typical panoramic radiographic feature of early ONJ [5, 9] and may represent an early imaging finding associated with bisphosphonate-induced ONJ (Figs. 8.1 and 8.2) [4, 5, 8, 9].

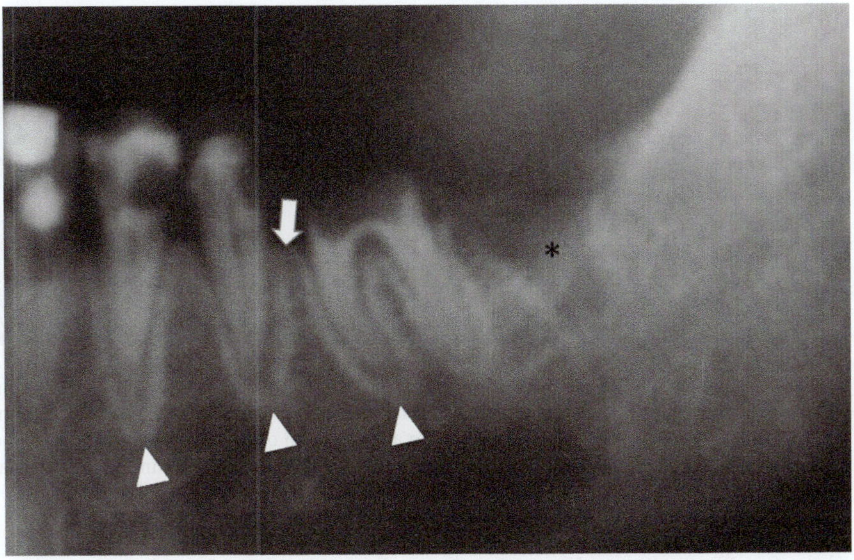

Fig. 8.1 Patient with a tooth extraction performed 1 year earlier. The focused panoramic view well demonstrates a persistent alveolar socket related to delayed socket healing (*). Note also the increased thickening of the alveolar lamina dura (*arrowheads*) and alveolar crest (*arrow*), as an early finding of osteonecrosis of the jaw (ONJ)

Several authors have described bone sclerosis as the most common finding: its appearance can range between subtle thickening of the lamina dura and alveolar crest (Fig. 8.1) to attenuated osteopetrosis-like sclerosis [4, 9, 10]. In advanced stages, osteonecrosis is seen as an irregular area of osteosclerosis with "a cotton wool-like'' appearance (Fig. 8.2b). Osteolyses often show a central sequestrum; lytic areas may also indicate foci of bacterial infection (Fig. 8.3) [4, 5, 9].

Periosteal reaction and bone sequestrum may be predominant in advanced stages of the disease (Fig. 8.4) [7, 9]. Pathologic fractures are a common finding, with one study showing fractures in 16 of 32 patients with ONJ [4, 5, 7, 9]. Narrowing of the marrow space and involvement of the inferior alveolar canal are also common findings at CT (Fig. 8.5) [4, 5, 9]. However, it was recently demonstrated that even if adjacent alveolar bone is altered by lytic or sclerotic changes, sparing of the mandibular canal may represent the diagnostic clue for malignancies [11, 12]. CT is a useful imaging modality to demonstrate both the size and the type of alveolar involvement, to precisely assess the dimensions and locations of the lesions, and to define lesion margins during management (Fig. 8.6) [11, 12]. If the maxilla is involved, there may be associated abnormalities in the adjacent maxillary sinus, from muco-periosteal thickening to air-fluid levels and purulent drainage (Fig. 8.7) [9, 11, 12].

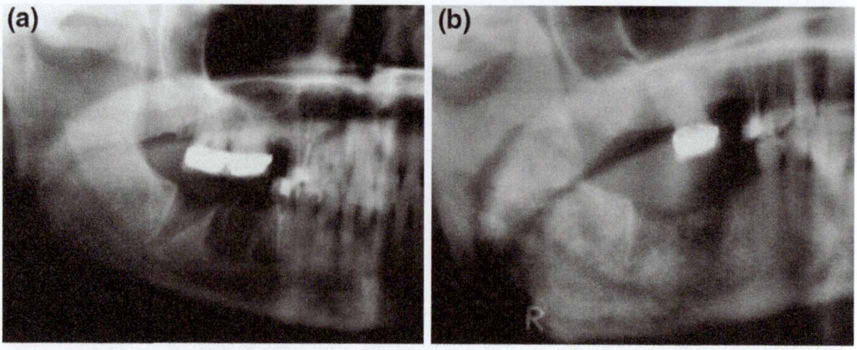

Fig. 8.2 Follow-up panoramic radiograph in a patient who underwent a tooth extraction. **a** Panoramic radiograph 1 month after extraction. **b** Panoramic radiograph 1 year after extraction. Delayed healing of the socket is readily visible in a comparison of the two images. Note also the thickened and disorganized medullary trabeculation, with cortical thickening and a typical "cotton-wool" appearance

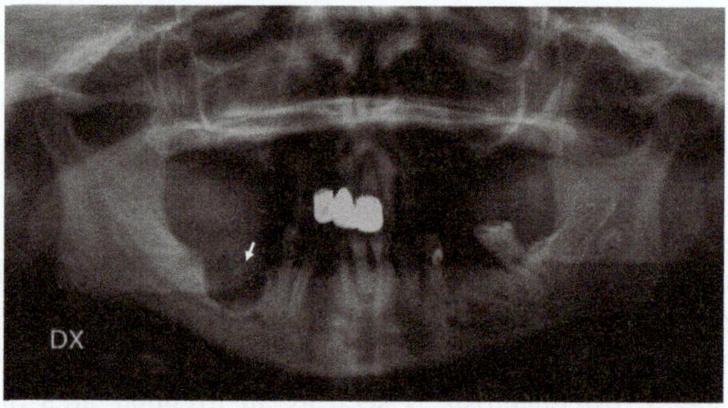

Fig. 8.3 Panoramic radiograph in a patient with ONJ showing a very large osteolytic area with central bone sequestrum (*arrow*)

8.3 Magnetic Resonance Imaging

In most cases, MRI is not used in the evaluation of a patient in whom ONJ is suspected, especially if the disease is in the early stage. However, as is the case with CT, disease extent is better demonstrated on MRI in the context of the clinical evaluation [9, 11–13]. The primary role of MRI is to assess the degree of bone and soft-tissue involvement, which may be helpful in planning surgical debridement in intractable cases not responding to conservative treatment [9, 14–16]. The signal-intensity changes on MRI encompass the bone and adjacent soft tissues, with variable signal-intensity abnormalities on T1- and T2-weighted images.

Typical ONJ findings on MRI are a decreased signal intensity on T1-weighted images and intermediate/high signal intensity on T2-weighted and/or short tau inversion-recovery (STIR) images, suggestive of edema and inflammation

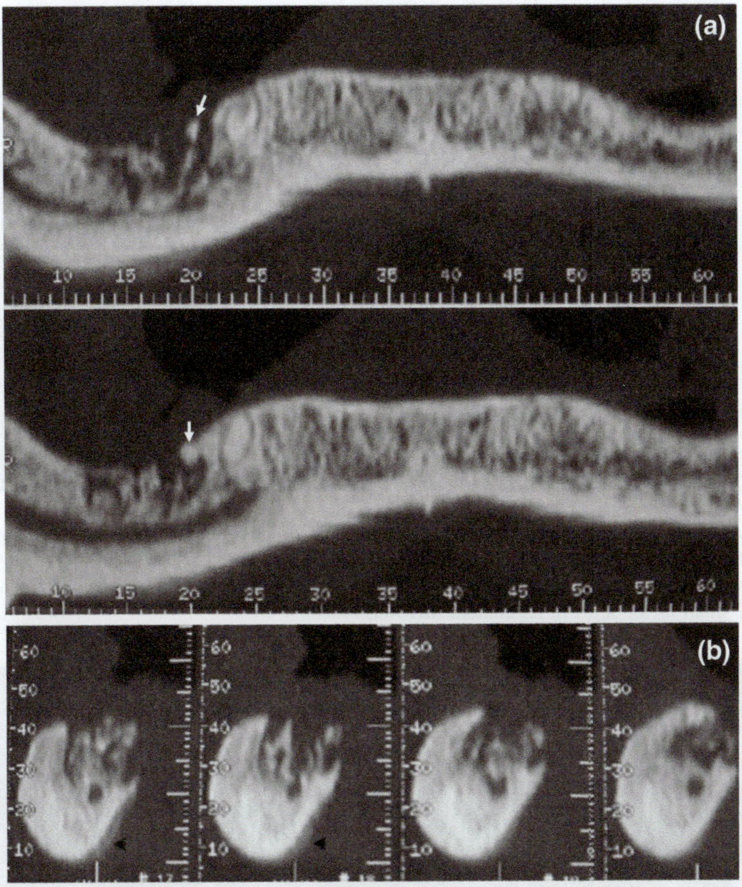

Fig. 8.4 CT Denta-scan. **a** Panoramic view shows lytic lesion in the right mandible with small sclerotic bone sequestra (*arrows*). **b** A thick and regular periosteal reaction (*arrowheads*) is well demonstrated on a cross-sectional image series

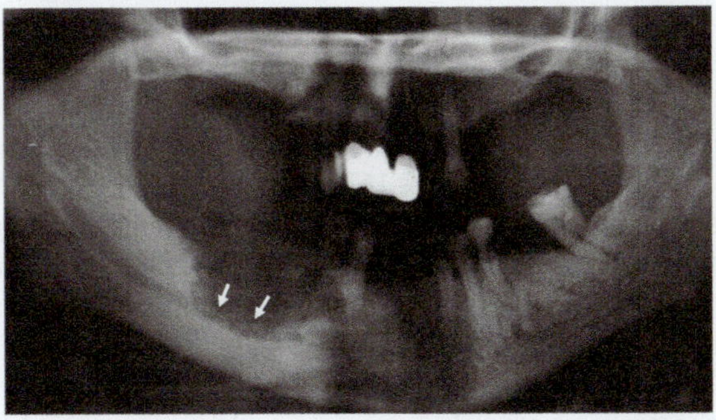

Fig. 8.5 Panoramic radiograph shows a wide osteolytic area involving the mandibular canal (*arrows*)

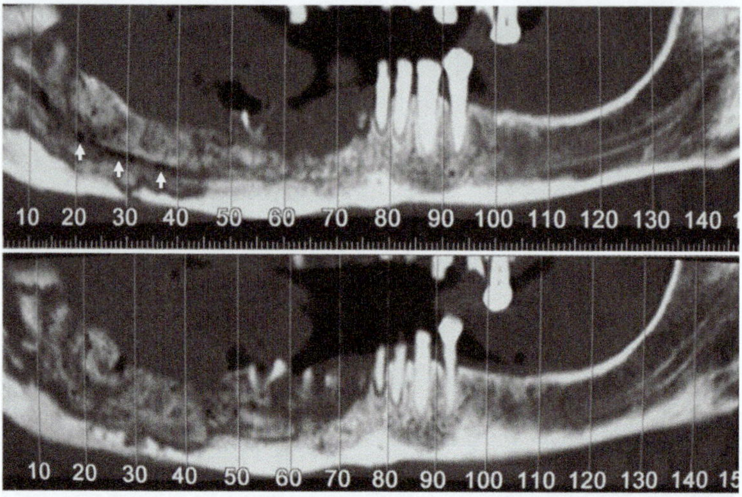

Fig. 8.6 CT Denta-scan. Two different panoramic views show the extensive involvement of the right mandible and the presence of both osteolytic and sclerotic foci, determining a mottled or "cotton-wool" appearance. Note also the involvement of the mandibular canal, evidenced by several small air bubbles in its content (*arrows*)

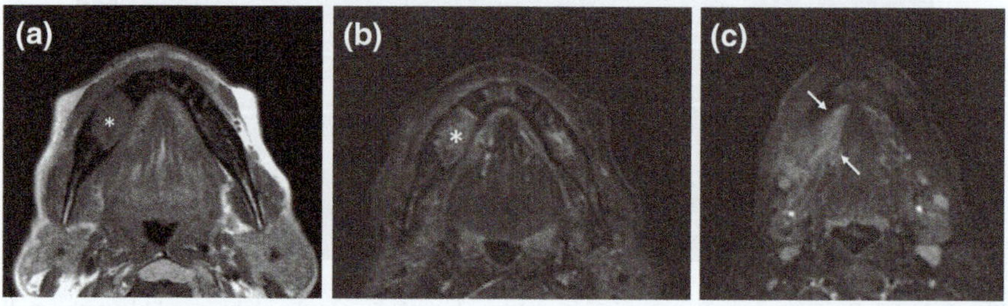

Fig. 8.7 MRI in a patient with ONJ-related osteonecrosis. **a** T1-weighted axial MRI shows a large hypointense lesion (*) involving the right mandible. **b** On axial STIR, the osteonecrotic focus is mildly hyperintense. **c** More caudal STIR MRI shows extensive involvement of the periosseous soft tissues

(Fig. 8.7a, b), with a variable degree of enhancement after the administration of contrast medium. Signal-intensity changes may be restricted to the cortex or extend to the bone marrow, adjacent soft tissues (Fig. 8.7c), maxillary sinus, and inferior alveolar canal [9, 13–16]. In cases of soft-tissue involvement, there is increased soft-tissue signal intensity on T2-weighted images (Fig. 8.7c) [9, 13–16]. However, signal-intensity changes on T2-weighted images and contrast enhancement findings may show enormous variability, due to fatty marrow replacement, bone sclerosis, or sequestrum [9, 13–18].

After gadolinium administration, the changes in signal intensity may be more extensive, suggesting greater disease extent than determined from the CT appearance of the involved bone (Fig. 8.8) [9, 13–16]. Bone marrow enhancement

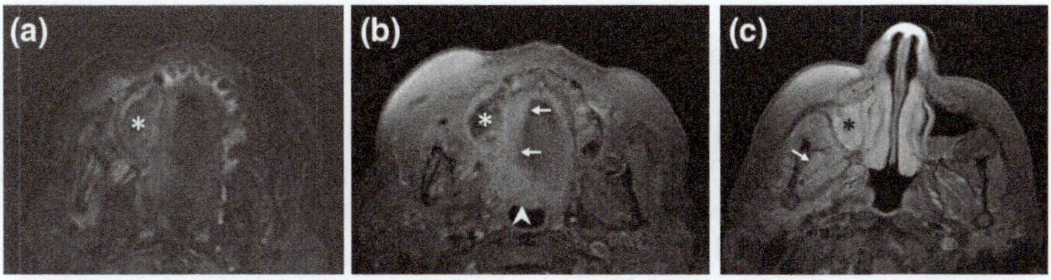

Fig. 8.8 MRI in a patient with maxillary osteonecrosis. **a** Axial STIR shows large osteonecrotic involvement (*) of the right maxillary bone. **b** Fat-suppressed T1-weighted axial MRI after gadolinium administration shows mild and diffuse enhancement around the osteonecrotic lesion (*) with involvement of the soft palate (*arrows*) and oropharyngeal wall (*arrowhead*). **c** More cranial fat-suppressed T1-weighted axial MRI after gadolinium administration shows thickening and enhancement of the maxillary sinus mucosa (*) as well as mild enhancement of the pterygoid muscles (*arrow*)

correlates with both the degree of fatty marrow replacement and a decrease in signal intensity on T1-weighted images [4] and typically spares the low T2 signal of the bone sequestrum [9, 13–18]. Soft-tissue enhancement is variable and may involve the mylohyoid ridge, buccinator muscle, orbicular muscle, maxillary sinus, and masticator space and muscles (Fig. 8.8) [9, 13–18]. There may be a focal mass-like thickening of these muscles, which clinically may mimic neoplastic involvement [19–21].

To date, only a few reports have described the MRI features of early-stage ONJ. According to Bisdas et al. [4], in early cases in which there are open wound areas and mild symptoms, decreased signal intensity on T1-weighted images is associated with intermediate or slightly increased signal intensity on T2-weighted images. At the periphery of wound lesions, there is usually a decrease in signal intensity on T2-weighted images [9].

In late stages or chronic cases, the signal intensity on T2-weighted images is also variable. Some authors have described decreased or mildly elevated signal intensity on T2-weighted images in patients with late or chronic stages of ONJ [9,13–16]. Nevertheless, the exact clinical stage of disease in the assessed patients was not clearly specified in these studies, which may explain the reported discrepancies in signal intensity on T2-weighted images [9, 13–18].

A correlation was noted between the patterns of signal-intensity changes and histologic findings [9, 17]. Areas with increased signal intensity on T2-weighted or STIR images were thought to correspond histologically to a chronic osteomyelitic pattern; areas with decreased signal intensity on T2-weighted or STIR images were histologically consistent with necrosis [9, 17].

Cervical lymphadenopathy is also a common finding associated with ONJ [9, 13–18]; it is most commonly submandibular, followed by the submandibular angle and jugulo-digastric chains [9, 13–18].

The sensitivity of MRI in the identification of ONJ varies between studies. Raje et al. [18] found MRI to be relatively insensitive in the assessment of ONJ relative to other anatomic and functional imaging modalities. They suggested that this difference was due to a lack of contrast material administration or to the predominance of study patients with advanced-stage disease. In a study by García-Ferrer et al. [14], MRI allowed the identification of all symptomatic lesions as well as additional lesions not appreciated at clinical examination. Finally, Bedogni et al. [17] described the MRI appearance of ONJ in patients with uncontrollable pain unresponsive to conventional treatment before surgical resection. In areas of exposed bone, decreased signal intensity on T2-weighted or STIR images was noted. Areas with unexposed bone demonstrated increased signal intensity on T2-weighted or STIR images, an appearance that may confirm that of unexposed lesions described in other imaging studies [9, 13–18].

8.4 Functional Imaging

Increased uptake at bone scintigraphy is noted in a majority (60–90%) of ONJ cases [6, 22]. Single-photon-emission CT (SPECT) and planar bone scintigraphy may allow differentiation between the decreased uptake of a sequestrum and the adjacent hyperactivity associated with reactive bone [6, 22]. It is unclear whether uptake occurs within the ONJ lesion or within surrounding reactive bone [6, 22]. Only a relatively small number of studies have evaluated the utility of fluorodeoxyglucose (FDG) positron emission tomography (PET) in the context of ONJ; however, FDG PET appears to be sensitive but not specific in this setting [22]. The increased FDG uptake associated with ONJ may be indicative of a healing response, inflammation, or infection at the site [6, 22].

8.5 Differential Diagnosis

Regarding the differential diagnosis in bisphosphonate-treated patients, metastatic disease in the jaws is a major concern [9]. The most common primary tumors are breast, kidney, prostate, lung, and stomach cancers, with metastases occurring four times more frequently in the mandible than in the maxilla. Metastatic bone changes seen at CT or MRI are similar to those caused by primary tumors of the jaws and may be localized or diffuse, lytic, or mixed [9, 13–18, 23, 24]. Lymphadenopathy may also be present, and in the presence of necrotic lymph nodes may support the diagnosis of metastatic disease. A very important, recently highlighted, diagnostic criterion to differentiate ONJ from metastases is sparing of the continuity of the mandibular canal cortex [9, 13–18, 23, 24]. Specifically, the cortex of the mandibular canal remains intact even though the adjacent alveolar bone shows lytic or sclerotic changes. This may represent a protective feature of the mandible during the pathological bone remodeling process [9, 13–18, 23, 24].

Osteomyelitis of the jaws is another important disease that should be differentiated from bisphosphonate-related lesions. Osteomyelitis may develop as a result of odontogenic infection, focal injury after tooth extraction, complicated fracture, or as the sequelae of immunocompromise (i.e., in patients with multiple myeloma). It may present as suppurative, sclerosing, tuberculous, or associated with periostitis [9, 13–18, 23, 24]. If the history does not include an acute onset with a severe systemic reaction suggesting a suppurative osteomyelitis, the diagnosis of chronic osteomyelitis may radiographically overlap with that of bisphosphonate-induced osteonecrosis. Moreover, the MRI appearance of osteomyelitis may depend on the patient's age and underlying medical conditions as well as the infecting organism [9, 13–18, 23, 24]. The bone marrow may initially have a normal appearance but low signal intensity in T1-weighted images and high signal intensity in T2-weighted images are sometimes present, with low intensity of the sequestrum on both T1- and T2-weighted images. Soft-tissue involvement is also common in osteomyelitis in which there is edema and abnormal enhancement of the soft tissue outside the infected areas, similar to bisphosphonate-induced osteonecrosis. Osteomyelitis can trigger a proliferative periosteal reaction or diffuse osteolytic changes with extension to the mandibular angle, ramus, or condyle and indistinct borders.

Osteoradionecrosis in irradiated patients leads to an increase in marrow space, which contains necrotic tissue, followed by sequestration with the typical "moth-eaten" appearance [23, 24].

Finally, another disease entity that can lead to osteonecrosis of the jaws is neuralgia-inducing cavitational osteonecrosis [25]. The dissolution of the alveolar medullary bone can cause loosening and, eventually, loss of the teeth; however, patients initially complain of severe and persistent atypical facial pain or trigeminal neuralgia. The affected bone is radiolucent with irregular borders.

8.6 Conclusions

Although the changes associated with ONJ are apparent with various imaging modalities, the findings are typically nonspecific. Currently, the primary role of imaging is to demonstrate the extent of disease before surgical intervention and complications such as pathologic fractures. The clinical implications of the imaging-based diagnosis of unexposed lesions that may be associated with bisphosphonate treatment are currently unknown. It is important for the radiologist to be aware of this entity and to include ONJ in the differential diagnosis in patients with a history of bisphosphonate treatment, so as to avoid unnecessary biopsies with potentially hazardous outcomes.

References

1. Estilo CL, Van Poznak CH, Wiliams T et al (2008) Osteonecrosis of the maxilla and mandible in patients with advanced cancer treated with bisphosphonate therapy. Oncologist 13:911–920
2. Ruggiero SL, Fantasia J, Carlson E (2006) Bisphosphonate-related osteonecrosis of the jaw: background and guidelines for diagnosis, staging and management. Oral Surg Oral Med Oral Pathol Oral Radiol Endod 102:433–441
3. Reid IR, Cundy T (2009) Osteonecrosis of the jaw. Skelet Radiol 38:5–9

4. Bisdas S, Chambron Pinho N, Smolarz A, Sader R, Vogl TJ, Mack MG (2008) Biphosphonate-induced osteonecrosis of the jaws: CT and MRI spectrum of findings in 32 patients. Clin Radiol 63:71–77
5. Stockmann P, Hinkmann FM, Lell MM et al (2010) Panoramic radiograph, computed tomography or magnetic resonance imaging. Which imaging technique should be preferred in bisphosphonate-associated osteonecrosis of the jaw? A prospective clinical study. Clin Oral Investig 14:311–317
6. Catalano L, Del Vecchio S, Petruzziello F et al (2007) Sestamibi and FDG-PET scans to support diagnosis of jaw osteonecrosis. Ann Hematol 86:415–423
7. Store G, Larheim TA (1999) Mandibular osteoradionecrosis: a comparison of computed tomography with panoramic panoramic radiography. Dentomaxillofac Radiol 28:295–300
8. Chiandussi S, Biasotto M, Dore F, Cavalli F, Cova MA, Di Lenarda R (2006) Clinical and diagnostic imaging of bisphosphonate-associated osteonecrosis of the jaws. Dentomaxillofac Radiol 35:236–243
9. Morag Y, Morag-Hezroni M, Jamadar DA et al (2009) Bisphosphonate-related osteonecrosis of the jaw: a pictorial review. Radiographics 29:1971–1984
10. Khosla S, Burr D, Cauley J et al (2007) Bisphosphonate- associated osteonecrosis of the jaw: report of a task force of the American Society for Bone and Mineral Research. J Bone Miner Res 22:1479–1491
11. Elad S, Gomori MJ, Ben-Ami N (2010) Bisphosphonate-related osteonecrosis of the jaw: clinical correlations with computerized tomography presentation. Clin Oral Investig 14:43–50
12. Phal PM, Myall RW, Assael LA, Weissman JL (2007) Imaging findings of bisphosphonate-associated osteonecrosis of the jaws. AJNR Am J Neuroradiol 28:1139–1145
13. Bianchi SD, Scoletta M, Cassione FB, Migliaretti G, Mozzati M (2007) Computerized tomographic findings in bisphosphonate-associated osteonecrosis of the jaw in patients with cancer. Oral Surg Oral Med Oral Pathol Oral Radiol Endod 104:249–258
14. García-Ferrer L, Bagán JV, Martínez-Sanjuan V et al (2008) MRI of mandibular osteonecrosis secondary to bisphosphonates. AJR Am J Roentgenol 190:949–955
15. Unger E, Moldofsky P, Gatenby R et al (1988) Diagnosis of osteomyelitis by MRI. AJR Am J Roentgenol 150:605–610
16. Chong J, Hinckley LK, Ginsberg LE (2000) Masticator space abnormalities associated with mandibular osteoradionecrosis: MR and CT findings in five patients. AJNR Am J Neuroradiol 21:175–178
17. Bedogni A, Blandamura S, Lokmic Z et al (2008) Bisphosphonate-associated jawbone osteonecrosis: a correlation between imaging techniques and histopathology. Oral Surg Oral Med Oral Pathol Oral Radiol Endod 105:358–364
18. Raje N, Woo SB, Hande K et al (2008) Clinical, radiographic, and biochemical characterization of multiple myeloma patients with osteonecrosis of the jaw. Clin Cancer Res 14:2387–2395
19. American Association of Oral, Maxillofacial Surgeons (2009) Position paper on bisphosphonate-related osteonecrosis of the jaw: 2009 update. American Association of Oral and Maxillofacial Surgeons, Rosemont
20. Wutzl A, Eisenmenger G, Hoffmann M et al (2006) Osteonecrosis of the jaws and bisphosphonate treatment in cancer patients. Wien Klin Wochenschr 118:473–478
21. Abu-Id MH, Warnke PH, Gottschalk J et al (2008) "Bisphossy jaws": high and low risk factors for bisphosphonate-induced osteonecrosis of the jaw. J Craniomaxillofac Surg 36: 95–103
22. Dore F, Filippi L, Biasotto M, Chiandussi S, Cavalli F, Di Lenarda R (2009) Bone scintigraphy and SPECT/CT of bisphosphonate-induced osteonecrosis of the jaw. J Nucl Med 50:30–35
23. Hishberg A, Leibovich P, Buchner A (1994) Metastatic tumors to the jawbones: an analysis of 390 cases. J Oral Pathol Med 23:337–341

24. Weber AL, Kaneda T, Scrivani SJ et al (2003) Jaw: cysts, tumors, and nontumorous lesions. In: Som PM, Curtin HD (eds) Head and neck imaging. Mosby, St Louis, pp 930–995
25. Bouquot JE, Roberts AM, Person P et al (1992) Neuralgia-inducing cavitational osteonecrosis (NICO): osteomyelitis in 224 jaw-bone samples from patients with facial neuralgia. Oral Surg Oral Med Oral Pathol 73:307–309

Microbiological Aspects of Osteonecrosis of the Jaw

9

Stefania Leuci, Marco Friscia and Michele Davide Mignogna

Abstract

BIONJ is generally defined by the presence of necrotic bone (sequestrum) in the oral cavity following the administration of a drug belonging to the category of bisphosphonates (BPs). In this clinical status, the infection of the exposed bone derives from the microbial flora of the oral cavity. The literature now increasingly contains reports invoking subclinical forms of BIONJ, suggesting that BIONJ occurs even in the absence of exposed bone, with nonspecific symptoms of pain, loose teeth not explained by periodontal disease, and intraoral fistula not explained by pulp necrosis. The pathogenesis of BIONJ may represent a microbial-biofilm-mediated infectious disease in the context of BP therapy. Accordingly, biofilms are a potential target for clinical therapy, with specific antibiofilm agents used in the treatment and prevention of BIONJ.

9.1 Introduction

Bisphosphonates-induced osteonecrosis of the jaws (BIONJ) is a pathological condition that, as its name implies, follows the administration of a drug belonging to the group of bisphosphonates (BPs). It is characterized by the exposure of maxillary and/or mandibular necrotic bone, based on the ability of BPs to inhibit osteoclastic activity, resulting in suppression of bone turnover and fostering the preservation of bone structure and mineralization [1]. It has also been proposed

M. D. Mignogna (✉)
Department of Odontostomatological Sciences, Oral Medicine Unit,
University of Naples "Federico II", Naples, Italy
e-mail: mignogna@unina.it

F. S. De Ponte (ed.), *Bisphosphonates and Osteonecrosis of the Jaw: A Multidisciplinary Approach*, DOI: 10.1007/978-88-470-2083-2_9,

that BPs have an anti-angiogenic effect as well, reducing blood flow and thus inducing bone cell necrosis and apoptosis [2, 3]. However, there are also alternative explanations, such as an "outside-in" process in which mucosal damage provides oral bacteria with access to the underlying bone, leading to bone infection and necrosis [4]. In this scenario, the soft-tissue toxicity of BPs is the trigger leading to mucosal and bone necrosis [5].

According to the AAOM, the three main risk factors for developing BIONJ are: drug-related (potency and duration of BP therapy), local factors (anatomy, inflammatory conditions, trauma), and demographic and systemic factors (age, sex, cancer, osteoporosis). To this list other factors must be added: long-term corticosteroids and immunosuppressive therapy, smoking, alcohol consumption, poor oral hygiene, concomitant autoimmune diseases, hematologic/thrombotic disorders, metabolic disorders, malignancies, and genetic factors [6–8].

9.2 Infection and Stage 0 Disease

The jaw bones, unlike the long bones, are in a special environment in that they are particularly vulnerable to both acute and chronic infections. These may arise or be further complicated by surgical procedures as well as masticatory trauma, both of which expose the bone to a bacteria-laden environment. Nonetheless, under normal circumstances, healing is rarely complicated by infection. Infection is now believed to play a pivotal role in this clinical problem.

BIONJ is generally defined by the presence of necrotic bone (sequestrum) in the oral cavity; in this clinical status, infection of the exposed bone derives from the microbial flora of the oral cavity. As evidenced by the literature, the concept of subclinical forms of BIONJ is increasing. More recently, Mawardi and colleagues suggested that BIONJ can occur even in the absence of exposed bone (stage 0) [9]. Similarly, a recent position paper of the AAOMS [6] included stage 0 in its modified classification. Stage 0 is defined as clinical nonspecific symptoms of pain, loose teeth not explained by periodontal disease, intraoral fistula not explained by pulp necrosis, and radiographic findings suggesting BIONJ. Subclinical osteonecrosis may remain stable until complicated by odontogenic or periodontal infection or mucosal and dentoalveolar traumatic events. The clinical appearance may be further complicated by impaired wound healing due to direct effects of BPs or to comorbidities in these patients [10].

Recent studies have shown bacterial colonization in jaw bones affected by BIONJ. In debris and granulation tissue, *Actinomyces* is especially prevalent [11–14], but other anaerobic species, such as *Eikenella*, *Peptostreptococcus*, and *Legionella*, as well as fungi [15]. Hansen et al. reported that *Actinomyces* occurs in the jaw bones of >90% of BIONJ patients, as determined from histological archive material [11]. In addition, these authors found pseudoepitheliomatous hyperplasia in the majority of the patients with BIONJ, with or without tooth extractions. Thus, it seems that pseudoepitheliomatous hyperplasia is a relatively common feature that reflects the mucosal disruption in actinomycosis.

9.2.1 The Specific Role of *Actinomyces*

When viewed on microscopic slides, *Actinomyces* have a very typical morphology: they tend to create a mass of filamentous bacteria that varies in color between the center and the periphery of the colony (the so-called sun-ray effect). PAS, Gram, and silver stains are typically positive [16]. In contrast to the unequivocal microscopic identification, the clinical significance of finding colonies compatible with *Actinomyces* in biopsy is often unclear, although their presence can be responsible for the prolongation of healing and an increased duration of antibiotic treatment. It is likely that an evaluation of the "bacterial load" (number and surface area of the bacterial colonies relative to the surface of the tissue) in the tissue will facilitate an assessment of the clinical course of the disease.

Actinomyces are commonly found in gingivodental crevices [17]. Moreover, it is well known that the initial step in the pathogenesis of actinomycosis is the disruption of the mucosal barrier, which leads to bacterial implantation in damaged tissue. The mucosal defects may be the result of a tooth extraction *in primis* or of surgical procedures that interrupt the integrity of mucosal surfaces. A diagnosis of actinomycosis should be made only if the clinical features of pain, sinus tracts, and sulfur granules are noted, either clinically or through histopathology [18].

On the other hand, superficial trauma is not the only portal of entrance for infectious agents: endodontal and periodontal infections may provide a conduit allowing bacteria to reach the bone in the absence of mucosal breakdown [19].

9.3 Biofilms and BIONJ

The role of infection in the pathogenesis of BIONJ is supported by evidence of microbial biofilms in the bones of these patients. The biofilms can be seen on scanning electron microscopy [20].

Indeed, biofilm theory has emerged to explain the etiology of the chronic infections typical of BIONJ. In most natural environments and in chronic bacterial infections, planktonic bacteria (free-floating, single-cell phenotype) generally exist only transiently, and usually as a minor population. Emerging evidence describes the bacterial populations comprising biofilms as predominantly polymicrobial, sessile, community-based aggregations embedded in a self-secreted matrix that provides numerous advantages for persistence in the face of environmental and host-challenges [21]. This thin layer of microorganisms is the biofilm and it constitutes the predominant phenotype of nearly all bacteria in their natural habitat, whether pathogenic or environmental. The biofilm provides a bulwark against environmental stressors and can include organisms from multiple kingdoms, as in the case of mixed bacterial–fungal biofilms. Furthermore, the resident bacterial community in a biofilm has added defenses and multiple mechanisms for survival, such as defenses against phagocytosis, UV-radiation, viral attack, shear stress, and dehydration, as well as against biocides, antibiotics, and host immunity.

The biofilm is considered a primitive form of cellular differentiation, with a primitive circulatory system, homeostasis, and "integrality," similar to eukaryotic tissues in their intercellular cooperation. The ability of bacterial cells to behave as a community is the result of complex intracellular and intercellular communication based on a signaling system regulated by quorum-sensing and response, two mechanisms that are ubiquitous in bacteria and which have been implicated in the regulation of very different and complex physiological processes, depending on the cellular density. The language used for this intercellular communication is based on small, self-generated signal molecules, known as bacterial pheromones, with different chemical structures (N-homoserine lactones and their derivatives in gram-negative and octapeptides and amino acids in gram-positive bacteria) [22]. Microbial biofilms are not just present on the bone surface exposed to the oral cavity but are also found in the deeper structure of the bone [12], which could account for the chronic infectious nature of BIONJ and at the same time could explain the resistance to current conventional therapeutic approaches.

Though epidemiologic evidence points to biofilms as a source of several chronic infectious diseases, the exact mechanisms by which biofilm-associated microorganisms elicit disease are poorly understood. Biofilm infections share clinical characteristics. They develop preferentially on inert surfaces or on dead tissue and occur commonly on medical devices and fragments of dead tissue such as the sequestra of dead bone seen in BIONJ. They can also form on living tissues, as in the case of endocarditis. Sessile bacterial cells release antigens and stimulate the production of antibodies; however, antibodies are not effective in killing bacteria within biofilms and may cause immune-complex-related damage to surrounding tissues. Even in individuals with excellent cellular and humoral immune reactions, biofilm infections are rarely resolved by host defense mechanisms [23]. Antibiotic therapy typically reverses the symptoms caused by planktonic cells released from the biofilm, but fails to kill the biofilm. The detachment of cells or cell aggregates, the production of endotoxin, increased resistance to the host immune system, and the provision of a niche for the generation of resistant organisms are all biofilm traits capable of initiating the disease process [24]. The resulting infection may go undectected for long periods, until it presents itself as exposed bone and is eventually diagnosed as what we now clinically describe as BIONJ.

The nature of biofilm structure and the physiological attributes of biofilm organisms confer an inherent resistance to antimicrobial agents, whether antibiotics, disinfectants, or germicides. One or more of the following mechanisms may be responsible for resistance: (i) delayed penetration of the antimicrobial agent through the biofilm matrix, (ii) altered growth rate of biofilm organisms, and (iii) other physiological changes due to the biofilm's mode of growth.

According to Koch's postulates, a causative relationship between a microorganism and a disease requires that: (i) the organism is regularly found in the lesions of the disease, (ii) it can be isolated in pure culture on artificial media, (iii) inoculation of this culture produces a similar disease in experimental animals, and (iv) the organism can be recovered from the lesions of these animals [25]. In 2009, Hall-Stoodley and Stoodley stated that in many cases biofilm infections cannot be proven according to Koch's postulates as the causative organism of BIONJ because of an absence of biofilm markers and of animal models to study the biofilm [26]. Nonetheless, the presence of microbial biofilms is well documented for dental caries and periodontitis [27] and it can be safely assumed that many of the cases of BIONJ described in the literature are characterized by preexisting dental infection [19].

In a recent published study [20], microbial biofilms in BIONJ were compared with those pertaining to osteomyelitis of the jaw. In all cases of BIONJ, multiple bacterial morphotypes were observed: short and long rods, cocci in clusters, and filamentous, crescent-shaped, and branching forms. Specifically, bacteria from the genera *Fusobacterium, Streptococcus, Actinomyces, Selenomonas*, and *Bacillus* were represented. These gram-positive and gram-negative organisms, including aerobes and anaerobes, are usually found in the oral cavity and often in association with odontogenic and periodontal infections. In addition, the authors observed fungal organisms consistent with *Candida albicans* colonizing the bone in all cases of BIONJ, often co-aggregating with bacterial biofilm organisms. By contrast, fungal organisms were not observed in any of the osteomyelitis specimens [20].

9.4 Conclusions

Despite the presence of these bacterial conglomerates in many patients with BIONJ, there is no clear evidence to answer the question whether infection is a primary or secondary event in BIONJ pathophysiology and whether it initially arises in the bone or soft tissue. In 2009, Silverman and Landesberg suggested that "inside-out" (matrix necrosis) and "outside-in" (biofilm colonization of exposed jaw bone) processes occur in tandem to produce the clinical appearance of BIONJ [15]. In both of these proposed mechanisms, the role of infection appears to be a critical step in the pathogenesis of BIONJ.

The clinical and microscopy findings in BIONJ described in the literature to date suggest the presence of a biofilm-mediated infectious process that must be prevented and treated, with many differences in bacterial morphotypes compared with osteomyelitis of the jaw occurring in the absence of BPs. It seems that the affected bone in BIONJ is more susceptible to bacterial and fungal colonization [20]. Ganguli et al. studied bacterial adhesion onto uncoated and BP-coated hydroxyapatite (HA) materials. They found that a significantly higher number of bacteria adherent to pamidronate-coated HA than to either uncoated HA (60-fold increase) or clodronate-coated HA (90-fold increase) [28]. These data provide new insight into the role of the relative potencies of the different types of BPs in the context of biofilm adhesion and behavior.

Currently, no universal and standardized therapeutic protocol has been approved for treating BIONJ. The few guidelines currently in use commonly suggest a conservative approach, made up systemic and topical antibiotic therapy and a preventive protocol to maintain good oral health. As a result, antibiotic treatment decisions are based on the collective clinical experience. It is not yet clear whether the discontinuation of BPs results in the improvement of osteonecrosis of the jaws [29].

New microbiological research and randomized controlled studies will better clarify the role of infection in the pathogenesis of BIONJ and encourage the development of new therapeutic strategies aimed at biofilm-specific targets. Since the treatment of BIONJ patients remains an enormous challenge, microbiological data could give clinicians a new way to look at BIONJ.

References

1. Almazrooa SA, Woo SB (2009) Bisphosphonate and nonbisphosphonate-associated osteonecrosis of the jaw: a review. J Am Dent Assoc 140:864–875
2. Fournier P, Boissier F, Filleur S et al (2002) Bisphosphonates inhibit angiogenesis in vitro and testosterone-stimulated vascular regrowth in the ventral prostate in castrated rats. Cancer Res 62:6538–6544
3. Santini D, Vincenzi B, Avvisati G et al (2002) Pamidronate induces modifications of circulating angiogenic factors in cancer patients. Clin Cancer Res 8:1080–1084
4. Hansen T, Kunkel M, Weber A et al (2006) Osteonecrosis of the jaws in patients treated with bisphosphonates: histomorphologic analysis in comparison with infected osteoradionecrosis. J Oral Pathol Med 35:155–160
5. Reid IR, Bolland MJ, Grey AB (2007) Is bisphosphonate-associated osteonecrosis of the jaw caused by soft tissue toxicity? Bone 41:318–320
6. Ruggiero SL, Dodson TB, Assael LA et al (2009) American Association of Oral and Maxillofacial Surgeons position paper on bisphosphonate-related osteonecrosis of the jaws—2009 update. J Oral Maxillofac Surg 67:2–12
7. Yoneda T, Hagino H, Sugimoto T et al (2010) Bisphosphonate-related osteonecrosis of the jaw: position paper from the Allied Task Force Committee of Japanese Society for Bone and Mineral Research, Japan Osteoporosis Society, Japanese Society of Periodontology, Japanese Society for Oral and Maxillofacial Radiology, and Japanese Society of Oral and Maxillofacial Surgeons. J Bone Miner Metab 28(4):365–383
8. Siddiqi A, Payne AG, Zafar S (2009) Bisphosphonate-induced osteonecrosis of the jaw: a medical enigma? Oral Surg Oral Med Oral Pathol Oral Radiol Endod 108:e1–e8
9. Mawardi H, Treister N, Richardson P et al (2009) Sinus tracts—an early sign of bisphosphonate-associated osteonecrosis of the jaws? J Oral Maxillofac Surg 67(3):593–601
10. Landesberg R, Cozin M, Cremers S et al (2008) Inhibition of oral mucosal cell wound healing by bisphosphonates. J Oral Maxillofac Surg 66(5):839–847
11. Hansen T, Kunkel M, Weber A et al (2006) Osteonecrosis of the jaws in patients treated with bisphosphonates—histomorphologic analysis in comparison with infected osteoradionecrosis. J Oral Pathol Med 35:155–160
12. Sedghizadeh PP, Kumar SK, Gorur A et al (2008) Identification of microbial biofilms in osteonecrosis of the jaws secondary to bisphosphonate therapy. J Oral Maxillofac Surg 66(4):767–775
13. Lugassy G, Shaham R, Nemets A et al (2004) Severe osteiomyelitis of the jaw in long-term survivors of multiple myeloma: a new clinical entity. Am J Med 117:440–441
14. Melo MD, Obeid G (2005) Osteonecrosis of the maxilla in a patient with a history of bisphosphonate therapy. J Can Dent Assoc 71:11–13
15. Silverman SL, Landesberg R (2009) Osteonecrosis of the jaw and the role of bisphosphonates: a critical review. Am J Med 122(Suppl 2):S33–S45
16. Goldberg MH (2003) Diagnosis and treatment of cervicofacial actinomycosis. Oral Maxillofac Surg Clin 15:51–58

17. Smego RA, Foglia G (1998) Actinomycosis. Clin Infect Dis 26:1255–1263
18. Russo TA (2005) Agents of actinomycosis. In: Mandell GL (ed) Douglas and Bennett's principles and practice of infectious diseases, 6th edn. Churchill Livingstone, New York, pp 2924–2934
19. Kumar KS, Gorur A, Schaudinn C et al (2010) The role of microbial biofilms in osteonecrosis of the jaw associated with bisphosphonate therapy. Curr Osteoporos Res 8:40–48
20. Sedghizadeh PP, Kumar SK, Gorur A et al (2009) Microbial biofilms in osteomyelitis of the jaw and osteonecrosis of the jaw secondary to bisphosphonate therapy. J Am Dent Assoc 140(10):1259–1265
21. Randall DW, Garth DE (2008) Biofilms and chronic infections. J Am Med Assoc 299(22):2682–2684
22. Lazăr V, Chifiriuc MC (2010) Architecture and physiology of microbial biofilms. Roum Arch Microbiol Immunol 69(2):95–107
23. Costerton JW, Stewart PS (1999) Bacterial biofilms: a common cause of persistent infections. Science 21(284):1318–1322
24. Donlan RM, Costerton JW (2002) Biofilms: survival mechanisms of clinically relevant microorganisms. Clin Microbiol Rev 15(2):167–193
25. Davis BD (1980) Evolution of microbiology and of microbes. In: Davis BD, Dulbecco R, Eisen HN, Ginsberg HS (eds) Microbiology, 3rd edn. Harper and Row, Philadelphia, p 7
26. Hall-Stoodley L, Stoodley P (2009) Evolving concepts in biofilm infections. Cell Microbiol 11(7):1034–1043
27. Siqueira JF Jr, Rôças I (2009) Community as the unit of pathogenicity: an emerging concept as to the microbial pathogenesis of apical periodontitis. Oral Surg Oral Med Oral Pathol Oral Radiol Endod 107(6):870–878
28. Ganguli A, Steward C, Butler SL et al (2005) Bacterial adhesion to bisphosphonate coated hydroxyapatite. J Mater Sci Mater Med 16(4):283–287
29. Rustemeyer J, Bremerich A (2010) Bisphosphonate-associated osteonecrosis of the jaw: what do we currently know? A survey of knowledge given in the recent literature. Clin Oral Investig 14:59–64

Prevention and the Role of the Dentist 10

Giacomo Oteri

Abstract

This chapter discusses and assesses the dentist's role in patients undergoing bisphosphonates (BPs) therapy. These drugs are potent inhibitors of bone resorption and bone remodeling due to their action on osteoclasts. Although they are widely used as part of the standard therapies for important pathologies, such as multiple myeloma, bone metastasis of solid cancers, and dismetabolic bone pathologies, their mechanism of action is not yet fully understood. Dental professionals are directly involved in the diagnosis and treatment of the unexpected side effects of BPs, necrotic manifestations of the jaws. Moreover, since oral surgical procedures are a key factor in developing osteonecrosis, the dentist has assumed a decisive role in its prevention. In this chapter, the risk factors and preventive measures in oncologic and osteoporotic patients are differentiated and clearly presented. The value of biochemical markers of bone activity in predicting the jaw osteonecrosis is also explained. The importance of the strict collaboration between dentist, oncologist, and physician is emphasized, including the need to adopt procedures that avoid unnecessary and invasive dental procedures, optimize oral health, and exclude local cofactors.

10.1 Introduction

Over the past two decades, intravenous amino bisphosphonates (NBPs), particularly pamidronate and zoledronic acid, have become the standard of care for the prevention and treatment of bone metastases from solid tumors and multiple

G. Oteri (✉)
Department of Dentistry, University of Messina, Messina, Italy
e-mail: giacomo.oteri@unime.it

F. S. De Ponte (ed.), *Bisphosphonates and Osteonecrosis of the Jaw: A Multidisciplinary Approach*, DOI: 10.1007/978-88-470-2083-2_10,

Table 10.1 Indications for use and dosage of amino-bisphosphonates and the relative potency of these agents (adapted from [1])

Bisphosphonate (Trade name, manufacturer)	Common indications for use	Dosage	Relative potency[a]
Etidronate (Didronel, P&G)	Paget's disease	300–750 mg/die × 6 months	1
Alendronate (Fosamax, Merck)	Osteoporosis	10 mg/day 70 mg/week	1,000
Risedronate (Actonel, P&G)	Osteoporosis	5 mg/day 35 mg/week	5,000
Ibandronate (Bonviva, Roche)	Osteoporosis	2.5 mg/day 150 mg/month	10,000
Pamidronate (Aredia, Novartis)	Bone metastases, Multiple myeloma	90 mg/3 weeks	100
Zoledronic acid (Zometa, Novartis)	Bone metastases, Multiple myeloma	4 mg/3 weeks	100.000
Zoledronic acid (Aclasta, Novartis)	Osteoporosis	5 mg/year	100.000

[a] Etidronate, a non-nitrogen-containing bisphosphonate is considered with relative potency of 1

myeloma (Table 10.1) [1, 2]. These drugs are prescribed as potent inhibitors of bone resorption and bone remodeling but, despite their widespread use, the mechanism of their action is not yet fully understood. NBPs inhibit enzymatic activities and osteoclast differentiation; at certain concentrations, they can limit angiogenesis and exert direct anti-tumoral effects [3–7]. The high affinity of pamidronate and zoledronic acid for hydroxyapatite is well established and explains their accumulation osteoclasts, with a dose-related effect. Due to the long half-lives of NBPs, they are able to reduce the bone resorption activity of these cells for several years [3]. Oral NBPs differ from the intravenous forms of these drugs in their specific concentrations and formulations. As anti-resorptive agents, they are effective in the treatment of metabolic bone diseases such as osteoporosis and osteopenia. Oral NBPs, such as alendronate, became available in 1995 and are prescribed world-wide [8, 9].

Until a few years ago, bisphosphonates were generally considered to be well tolerated, with minimal adverse effects. Prior to 2003, they were far removed from the concerns of dentists and oral and maxillofacial surgeons; however, in that year a side effect of NBP treatment, later referred to as bisphosphonates-induced osteonecrosis of the jaw (BIONJ), was documented and has since frequently been reported [10–14]. BIONJ is defined as the presence of exposed bone in the oral cavity that does not regress within 8 weeks in patients who are currently being treated or who were previously treated with systemic intravenous or oral NBPs and who have not undergone radiation therapy to the maxillofacial region. BIONJ can seriously affect the quality of life by producing significant degrees of morbidity [15]. Estimates of the cumulative incidence of BIONJ in cancer patients receiving i.v. BP range from 0.8 to 18.6% [15, 16]. The frequency of BIONJ in osteoporotic patients is between 0.01 and 0.04%. In the group of patients on NBPs who have undergone dental extractions, the frequency in the range of 0.09–0.34% [13, 14]. It is therefore of critical importance that dentists be aware of their role in the early diagnosis of osteonecrosis, its prevention, and the treatment options. In addition, a profound knowledge of the clinical recommendations is needed in order to advise patients on NBPs regarding appropriate dental treatment.

The role of the dentist can be summarized as follows:

1. Be aware of the risk of dento-alveolar surgical procedures in the development of BIONJ.
2. Recognize the clinical and radiographic features of osteonecrosis.
3. Identify the local and systemic risk factors in patients on NBPs that place them into the low- or high-risk group for BIONJ.
4. Adopt preventive strategies in patients on NBPs, and especially in those who require dento-alveolar surgical procedures.
5. Consider the predictive value of biochemical markers of metabolic bone activity in determining the risk of BIONJ.

10.2 Diagnostic Considerations

Since the publication of the first case series, it has been clear that the location and function of the maxillary bones explained their vulnerability to BIONJ. In fact, the majority of BIONJ cases involve patients who have undergone invasive dental procedures such as dento-alveolar, periapical, periodontal, or implant surgery. BIONJ exclusive effects on the mandible and maxilla are due to the fact that bisphosphonates become highly concentrated in these metabolically active bones [17]. The bones of the jaw have a higher blood supply than other bones in the body and a higher rate of bone turnover, and thus higher osteoclast activity. In addition, chronic dental disease, invasive dento-alveolar treatments, and the thin mucosal barrier protecting the bones of the jaw explain why BIONJ is manifested exclusively in the oral cavity [18].

In daily practice, it is well known that patients frequently do not inform the dentist of the drugs they are currently taking or medications that they took in the past which have since been discontinued. Thus, before a patient undergoes oral surgery, it is essential that the dentist ask the patient whether he/she suffers from any pathological bone syndromes that are or might be treated with NBPs. These, obviously, include metabolic bone disease (osteoporosis, osteopenia, Paget's disease), bone metastasis of solid tumors, and multiple myeloma. In addition to the NBP formulation, the dosage, frequency, and duration must be registered in the patient's medical record, as they are critical factors that may contribute to the development of osteonecrosis. Moreover, and particularly in the case of elderly or cancer patients, a detailed pharmacological history is essential and may require that the dentist communicate with the patient's health care practitioners (physician,

Table 10.2 Clinical staging scheme for the diagnosis of BIONJ according to the AAOMS (2008)

Staging	Clinical features
Stage 0	Regional or diffuse osteosclerosis in clinically symptomatic areas, dense confluence of cortical and cancellous bone, prominence of the inferior alveolar nerve canal, markedly thickened and sclerotic lamina dura
Stage 1	Cortical disruption, lack of bone fill after extraction and non-healing alveolar socket
Stage 2	Enlarged osteolytic areas in symptomatic patients
Stage 3	Bone sequestrum, pathologic fracture, oral-antral/oral-nasal communication, osteolysis extending to the inferior border of the mandible or sinus floor

family practitioner, gynecologist, endocrinologist, oncologist) who may be prescribing NBPs [19].

10.3 Clinical and Radiographic Features of BIONJ

It is mandatory for the dentist to recognize the signs and symptoms of BIONJ as an emergent maxillary disease. A clinical staging scheme, proposed by the American Association of Oral and Maxillofacial Surgeons (AAOMS), serves as the current clinical guidelines for the diagnosis of BIONJ (Table 10.2) [15]. These guidelines consist of five stages. Stage 1 is the "patient at risk", which refers to asymptomatic patients, i.e., without bone exposure, who have been treated with NBPs. Stages 0–3 describe the features of necrotic bone exposure, from early to advanced, and the association with pain, infection, fistula, and fracture. In patients with stage 0 disease, there is discomfort and non-specific oral symptoms without apparent exposure of necrotic bone. The first clinically evident sign of BIONJ is single or multifocal exposed necrotic bone in the jaws. The process is more common in the mandible, but, alone or in combination, may involve the maxilla too (Fig. 10.1).

Although most cases of exposed necrotic bone are the consequence of unsuccessful healing of alveolar bone after tooth extraction, patients wearing a denture or with mandibular or palatal tori covered with a thin mucosa are also at risk. In such cases, a non-healing mucosal breach, e.g., due to an unstable denture or small traumatic injury, could be a portal for oral bacteria to access the bones of the jaw (Figs. 10.2, 10.3). While the exposed necrotic bone is not painful in itself, the onset of a secondary infection will cause pain and may lead to cellulitis and abscess formation (Fig. 10.4). The differential diagnosis includes inflammatory, reactive, cystic and neoplastic pathologies that can involve the jaws.

Pathological fractures can occur in BIONJ and may go unrecognized as such if debridement surgeries have reduced the structural integrity of the mandible (Fig. 10.5). Other symptoms of BIONJ are oral-cutaneous, oral-antral, and oral-nasal fistulas, which appear in the advanced stages (Fig. 10.6).

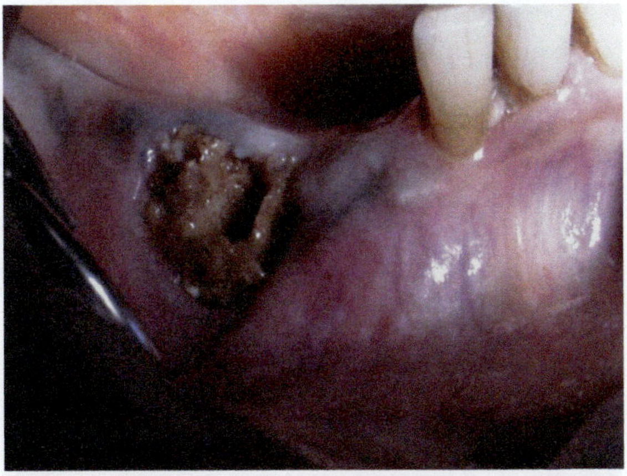

Fig. 10.1 Stage I BIONJ consequent to molar extraction

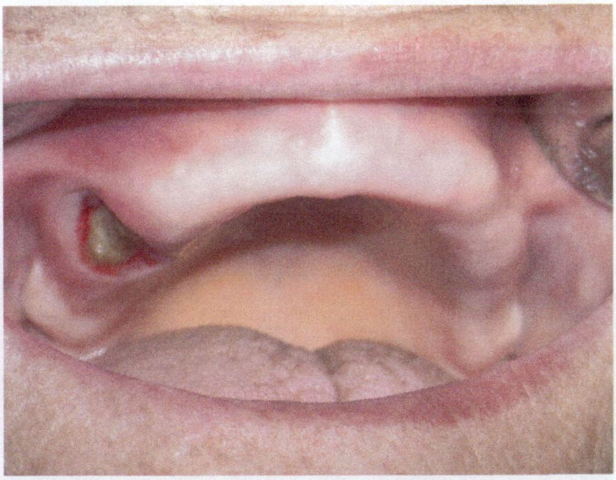

Fig. 10.2 Stage I: Maxillary exposure in a denture wearing patient

The radiologic features of the early stages of BIONJ illustrate the increasing bone mineral density that follows inhibition of osteoclast activity and proliferation (Fig. 10.7). In the exposed bone, the progressing osteonecrosis together with secondary infection results in focal areas of demineralization that may lead to the formation of a sequestrum (Figs. 10.8, 10.9).

10.4 Risk Factors in the Development of BIONJ

A risk assessment of BIONJ is strongly recommended in patients taking NBPs who require invasive dental procedures [20]. High-risk patients are those receiving high-dose and high-potency NBPs as chemotherapeutic agents. In this group, the

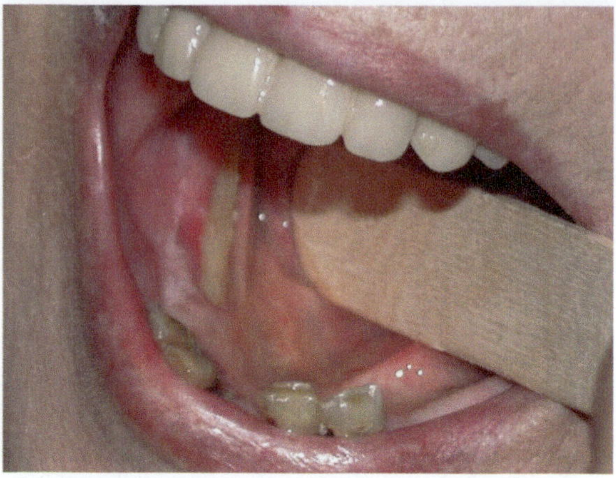

Fig. 10.3 Mandibular exposure associated with thin mucosal coverage

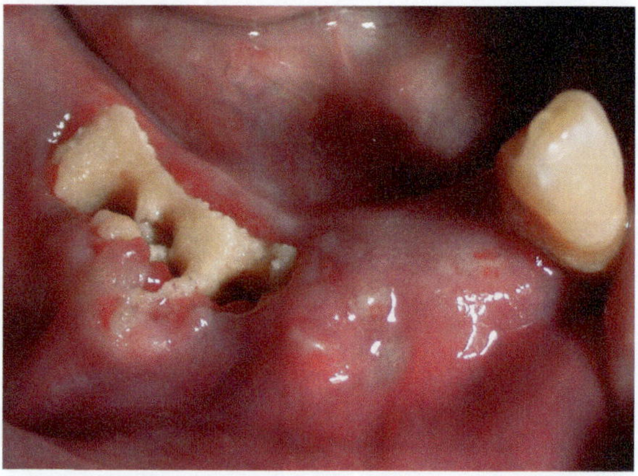

Fig. 10.4 Stage II: BIONJ consequent to teeth extraction

route of administration may consist of monthly treatment with high intravenous doses of pamidronate or zoledronic acid, or oral bisphosphonates, e.g., ibandronate, (Bondronat, Roche) 50 mg/day. Patients in the low-risk group are those on bisphosphonates for the treatment of osteoporosis, osteopenia, and Paget's disease. These patients typically receive 5 mg zoledronate (Aclasta Novartis)/year or 3 mg ibandronate (Bonviva, Roche)/3 months.

In both groups of patients, the inability of soft tissues to envelop the extraction socket—as may occur in patients undergoing extraction procedures without any preventive measures—results in exposure of the underlying bone and consequent infection. The final effect is a progressive necrotizing, unremitting osteomyelitis. Oral NBPs for osteoporosis treatment produce milder BIONJ than intravenous

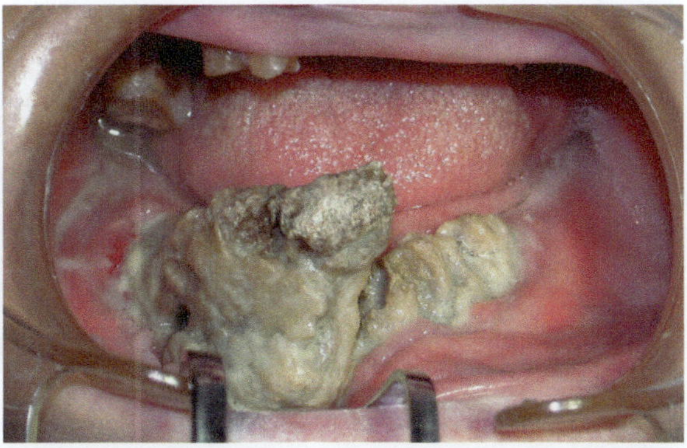

Fig. 10.5 Stage III: Pathological mandibular fracture of the symphysis

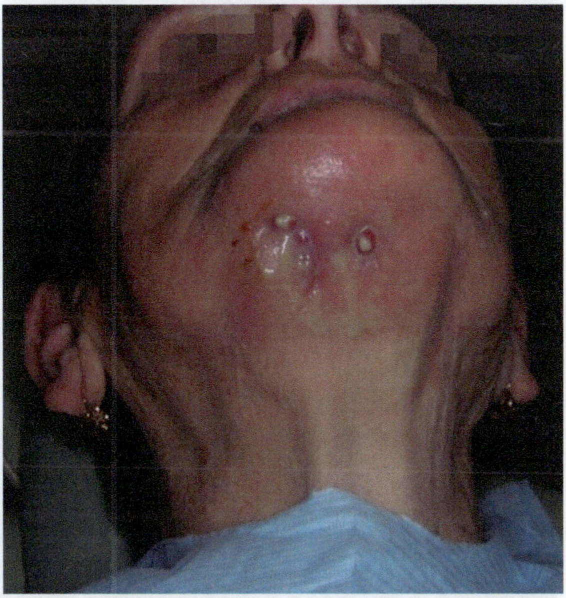

Fig. 10.6 Stage III: Oral cutaneous fistula in a patient with stage III disease

forms of these drugs since the degree of necrosis is related to the potency and dosage of NBPs. For metastatic cancer, the dose is 4–12 times higher than for osteoporosis [21]. Another factor that must be considered are differences in the mean period of BIONJ onset in patients on NBPs: typically, 9 months for zoledronate and 30–52 months for alendronate [22].

Moreover a relevant number of secondary local and general risk factors have been identified. The addition of secondary factors can potentially shift a patient from a low to a high risk of developing of BIONJ. These local risk factors include:

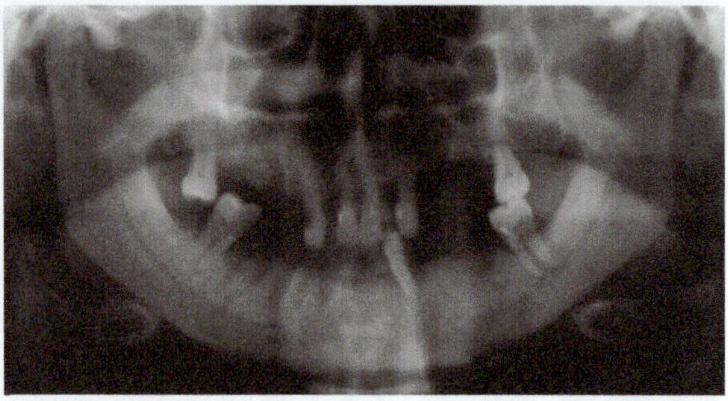

Fig. 10.7 Non-healing alveolar socket in patient with necrotic exposed bone

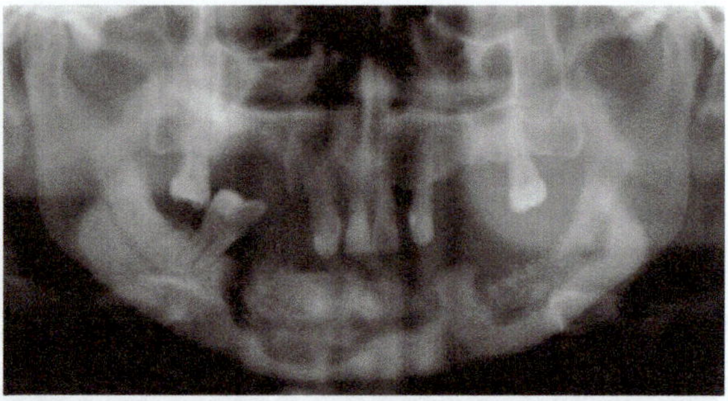

Fig. 10.8 Mandibular bone sequestra

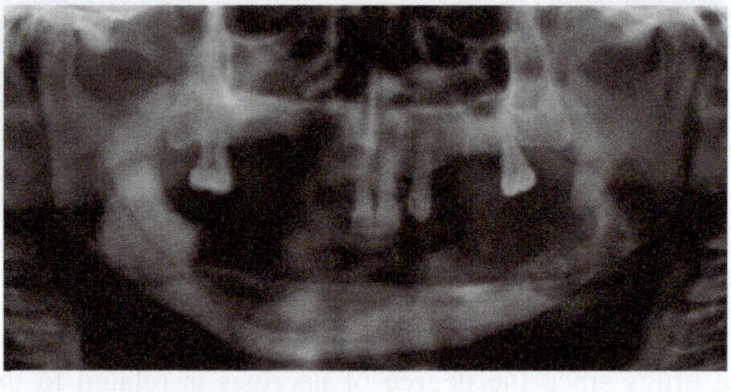

Fig. 10.9 Mandibular pathologic fracture

- All invasive dental procedures (16- to 44-fold higher risk)
- Extractions of the lower molars (more than two-thirds of BIONJ cases are mandibular)
- Trauma related to unstable dentures (5-fold higher risk)
- Thin mucosal coverage of the bones of the jaws [22, 23]

The role of periodontal and periapical diseases is not clear. Hoff et al. reported that cancer patients with a history of periodontal and dental abscesses have a seven-fold higher risk of BIONJ [25]. This was refuted in other studies, especially when oral surgery was avoided in these patients [24, 26].

The general risk factors involved in BIONJ are:

- Demographics (age > 60 years): Since blood circulation and the ability to recover from trauma are decreased in older patients, advanced age is considered to place patients at increased risk.
- Female gender. Women are at higher risk because they are more likely to receive NBPs, i.e., for the treatment of osteoporosis [27].
- Other drugs. Concomitant therapy with corticosteroids, chemotherapeutics, or thalidomide increases the risk of BIONJ because the molecular mechanisms of these medications include inflammatory and immune suppression involving osteoclasts, osteoblasts, and osteocytes, thus increasing the risk of osteonecrosis, although this issue is debated in the literature [28].
- Concomitant disease: Immunocompromise and uncontrolled diabetes are systemic conditions that can affect bone turnover.
- Life-style related: Heavy tobacco consumption and poor oral hygiene are associated with the delayed healing of surgical wounds and extraction sockets [29].
- Genetic factors: Single-nucleotide polymorphisms in the CYP2C8 gene influence the development of BIONJ in patients with multiple myeloma treated with NBPs [30].

Some of the above-mentioned risk factors can be eliminated or altered in patients on NBPs. Thus, for example, it is fundamental to encourage patients to stop smoking and to improve oral hygiene. If the patient's systemic condition permits the discontinuation of corticosteroid treatment or the completion of chemotherapy, then the dental invasive procedure can be delayed to reduce the risk of BIONJ.

10.5 Preventive Measures in Oncologic Patients

Given the ineffectiveness of currently available BIONJ treatments, prevention of the precipitating dental risk factors, especially in cancer patients, seems to be the most rational approach [31, 32]. As noted above, based on the oncologist's assessment, if the patient's clinical condition allows the postponement of NBP therapy, the dentist then assumes a decisive role. He or she has to carry out a complete dental screening to identify the presence of: odontogenic infections, compromised teeth that require intervention, periodontal disease, unstable dentures, and in limited cases, extraction. All patients need instructions on adequate hygiene control. At this point, all endodontic, conservative, and periodontal procedures should be performed. During and after medical treatment with intravenous NBPs, patients should not undergo any dental procedure without first consulting the treating physician [17, 33]. The administration of bisphosphonates by the oncologist can begin 6–8 weeks after the invasive procedure, when complete soft-tissue healing has been documented.

Three studies on the cost effectiveness of these preventive measures demonstrated that the development of BIONJ can be reduced by as much as 50–75% [34–36]. However, due to the very long lasting effects of bisphosphonates in bone, the discontinuation of intravenous NBPs offers no short-term benefits and does not seem to modify the risk of BIONJ following an invasive procedure. If systemic conditions permit, long-term discontinuation of NBPs might stabilize established sites of BIONJ, reduce the risk of new site development, and mitigate clinical symptoms.

According to current clinical recommendations, tooth extraction is absolutely contraindicated in high-risk NBP patients. Dental infections are to be treated with endodontic or periodontal procedures or medically "controlled" with long-term antibiotics. However, in teeth hopelessly destroyed by caries or in cases of root fracture or advanced periodontitis, conservative approaches may not be adequate; in fact, dental or periodontal abscesses increase the risk of BIONJ development [37].

Recently, preventive protocols for dental surgical extractions in high-risk patients were proposed. Lodi et al. treated 23 patients with 38 surgical extractions, all of them performed using a full-thickness mucoperiostal flap sutured coronally to close the alveolar socket. Three weeks before the extraction, the patients were instructed as follows: (a) professional oral hygiene and chlorhexidine (0.2%) mouth rinses once a day; (b) antibiotic therapy with 1 g amoxicillin/8 h starting 3 days before surgery and continuing until 14 days after surgery. The mean follow-up was 229.5 days and no apparent BIONJ was observed at 36 months [38].

Saia et al. also surgically treated 60 high-risk patients requiring dental extraction. These patients were given a cycle of antibiotic therapy consisting of amoxicillin, clavulanic acid, and metronidazole for 7 days. After surgery, the patients discontinued NBP therapy for one month. The authors reported that BIONJ occurred in only five patients, mostly in association with odontogenic osteomyelitis. They concluded that surgical closure of the sockets, antibiotic therapy, and a reduced concentration of NBPs favored healing in the socket and in alveolar bone. The improved results obtained with these protocols compared to simple tooth extraction can be ascribed to the fact that the alveolar socket is thus protected from exposure to oral pathogens, which may initiate bone infection and BIONJ. However, the efficacy and safety of surgical vs. simple tooth extraction protocols must be confirmed in further randomized controlled clinical trials [39].

10.6 Preventive Measures in Osteoporosis Patients

To date, there have been very few cases of BIONJ in patients taking oral NBPs. A survey by the AAOMS reported one new case of BIONJ for every 27,000 prescriptions of oral biphosphonates. Osteonecrosis resulting from oral NBPs preferentially involves the mandible. The majority of cases do not proceed past stage 3, with improvement or recovery in response to therapy [40, 41].

Like intravenous NBPs, oral NBPs increase the risk of BIONJ in patients undergoing tooth extraction, with an 8-fold higher risk linked to oral NBP use [42]. However, no cases of osteonecrosis as a result of routine dental procedures in patients taking oral NBPs have been described. Thus, the best preventive procedures are to avoid unnecessary and invasive dental procedures, to optimize oral health care, and to exclude local BIONJ risk cofactors.

Although elective dentoalveolar surgery does not appear to be contraindicated in this group, patients must still be informed of the risk of compromised bone healing. Given that delayed remodeling and healing in the post-extraction socket may be expected, patients might be advised to undergo surgical extractions with alveoloplasty and socket closure with a coronally sutured flap.

Since the very long lasting effects of bisphosphonates in bone are well known, temporary discontinuation of oral NBPs (drug holiday) in patients requiring oral surgery procedures has been recommended by several expert panels to reduce the risk of BIONJ. The safety of oral NBP interruption was demonstrated in a prospective and randomized clinical trial. A drug holiday after 5 years of NBP treatment did not increase the risk of non-vertebral fracture [43]. Whether a drug holiday reduces the risk of BIONJ associated with dental intervention has not been established, but the AAOMS has endorsed the following prudent guidelines based on the expert opinions of experienced surgeons:

- *Patients who have been under oral bisphosphonates for fewer than 3 years and have no clinical risk factors*: No alteration or delay in the planned oral surgery is necessary. "Ad hoc" informed consent should be provided if dental implants are placed (related to possible future implant failure and osteonecrosis of the jaws if the patient continues on oral bisphosphonates).
- *Patients who have been under oral bisphosphonates for fewer than 3 years who have taken an oral and have also taken corticosteroids concomitantly.*
- *Patients who have taken an oral bisphosphonate for more than 3 years with or without any concomitant prednisone or other steroid medication.*

In either of these circumstances, the prescribing physician should be contacted to consider, if systemic conditions permit, that the oral bisphosphonate be discontinued for at least 3 months before oral surgery and not restarted until osseous healing has occurred.

An interesting question refers to implant placement. Some retrospective studies declared that no BIONJ manifested after implant placement in patients taking NBPs [44, 45]. In patients under long-term NBP therapy for osteoporosis or in patients with concomitant steroid treatment, additional testing or alternative treatment options should be considered before implant surgery is performed. To date, only ten cases of BIONJ have been reported in patients who received an implant and were taking NBPs for osteoporosis. Despite this low risk in oral NBP users, their long-term prognosis remains uncertain. Therefore the potential risk of implant failure and BIONJ development and the need to maintain efficient long-term oral hygiene around the implant-supported prostheses must be clearly explained before the implant procedure [46].

10.7 Value of Biochemical Markers of Metabolic Bone Activity

It is clear that a causative role in BIONJ is played by dento-alveolar surgery. Dental extractions are the trigger in about the 86% of such cases, followed by oral surgery procedures and implant placements. As noted above, the treatment of BIONJ, especially in patients who have received intravenous NBPs, is thus far mainly palliative and efforts have instead been aimed at prevention, specifically, at identifying the biological parameters able to predict which patients are at high risk of developing BIONJ.

Rosen [47] proposed CTX (C-terminal cross-linking telopeptide of type I collagen) as a biological index of bone remodeling and resorption (Fig. 10.10). CTX is a specific breakdown product of type I collagen, which is the main structural organic component of bone and accounts for 98% of the total protein in bone. During bone resorption, the telopeptide fragment CTX is cleaved from the C-terminal of the main cross-linked chains of collagen by osteoclasts. Serum CTX levels are therefore proportional to the amount of osteoclastic resorption occurring at the time the blood sample was obtained. They can be measured in a simple automated blood test that requires a small blood sample taken in the morning, because of diurnal variation, from a fasted patient. In patients not taking bisphosphonates, normal values are usually 400–550 pg/ml. Lower values are indicative of varying degrees of suppression of normal bone turnover, such as during NBP treatment [47].

Marx was the first of several authors who introduced, in pilot studies, morning fasting serum CTX as a clinical tool to assess the risk of BIONJ, guide the clinician's evaluations of nonsurgical treatment response, and determine when oral surgery can be accomplished with the least risk. The test was evaluated in BIONJ patients either receiving intravenous bisphosphonates for bone cancer and multiple myeloma or taking oral bisphosphonates for osteoporosis. Low CTX values ($\leq$120 pg/ml) were found to reflect varying degrees of suppression of normal bone turnover. A clear distinction between oral and intravenous bisphosphonate patients was observed upon discontinuation of therapy (drug holiday). A 6 month drug discontinuation of oral bisphosphonates resulted in an improvement in CTX values that was related to: spontaneous resolution of the exposed bone, improvement in the amount of bone exposure, and evidence of a good healing response after surgery. These findings demonstrated that the discontinuation of oral NBPs can lead to a recovery of the functioning osteoclast population and to the re-establishment of osteoclast precursors in the bone marrow. However, in local debridement surgery, no improvement or response was observed following the discontinuation of intravenous bisphosphonates by oncologic patients.

The results confirm that bisphosphonate accumulation in bone is both greater and longer lasting with intravenous than with oral bisphosphonates. Moreover, there is atrophy of the osteoclast precursors in bone marrow such that the exhausted osteoclast population is unable to recover.

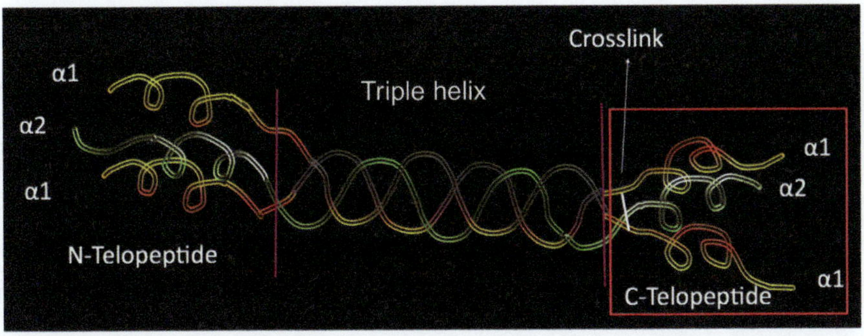

Fig. 10.10 Chains of collagen I

Marx suggested the following guidelines regarding serum CTX levels to evaluate the risk of BIONJ after surgical procedures in patients taking oral bisphosphonates [40]:
CTX >150 pg/ml:low risk.
CTX 100–150 pg/ml: moderate risk.
CTX ≤100 pg/ml; high risk.

Nonetheless, there is extensive scientific debate on serum CTX values as a predicting index of BIONJ risk. Some authors are of the opinion that, although the CTX test is not predictive of BIONJ development in an individual patient, it could still be useful to identify a "risk zone," with a cut- off value of <150–200 pg/ml. Based on this value, the oral bisphosphonate could be withdrawn until the patient is out of the CTX-defined "risk zone" [48–50]. However, other authors have claimed CTX measurements are of limited value in informing patient care and instead warrant continued investigation as well as the identification of other biomarkers [51, 52, 53].

10.8 Concluding Remarks

Differences in the incidence and clinical manifestations of BIONJ are conditioned by NBP potency, dose, and duration of therapy as well as precipitating local factors. Currently, BIONJ remains without defined treatment protocols and with an uncertain prognosis. Dental interventions necessitating the exposure alveolar bone should be avoided in cancer patients taking NBPs, but routine dental procedures are safe and can improve the patient's quality of life. The utility of bone-marker turnover testing as a tool for assessing the risk of BIONJ has yet to be clearly demonstrated. The discontinuation of NBP medications in osteoporotic patients undergoing dental extractions seems practical. If a NBP drug holiday is proposed, the dentist must evaluate the costs/benefits of the interruption, considering the important actions of these drugs in reducing osteoporotic fractures. Dental professionals will certainly welcome any measures that limit the risks of BIONJ and improve the treatment of these patients.

References

1. Hillner BE, Ingle JN, Berenson JR et al (2000) American Society of Clinical Oncology guideline on the role of bisphosphonates in breast cancer. J Clin Oncol 18:1378
2. Aapro M, Abrahamsson PA, Body JJ, Coleman RE, Colomer R, Costa L et al (2008) Guidance on the use of bisphosphonates in solid tumours: recommendations of an international expert panel. Ann Oncol 19:420–432
3. Kimmel DB (2007) Mechanism of action, pharmacokinetic and pharmacodynamic profile, and clinical applications of nitrogen containing bisphosphonates. J Dent Res 86:1022
4. Allegra A, Oteri G, Nastro Siniscalchi R, Alonci A (2007) Patients with bisphosphonates-associated osteonecrosis of the jaw have reduced circulating endothelial cells. Hematol Oncol 25(4):164–169
5. Alonci A, Allegra A, Bellomo G, Oteri G et al (2007) Patients with bisphosphonates associated osteonecrosis of the jaw have unmodified levels of soluble vascular endothelial growth factor receptor 1. Leuk Limphoma 48(9):1852–1854
6. Oteri G, Allegra A, Bellomo G, Alonci A et al (2008) Reduced serum levels of interleukin 17 in patients with osteonecrosis of the jaw in multiple myeloma subjects after bisphosphonates administration. Cytokine 43(2):103–104
7. Santini D, Vincenzi B, Hannon RA et al (2006) Changes in bone resorption and vascular endothelial growth factor after a single zoledronic acid infusion in cancer patients with bone metastases from solid tumours. Oncol Rep 15:1351
8. Delmas PD (2005) The use of bisphosphonates in the treatment of osteoporosis. Curr Opin Rheumatol 17:462
9. Kanis JA, Gertz BJ, Singer F et al (1995) Rationale for the use of alendronate in osteoporosis. Osteoporos Int 5:1
10. Marx RE (2003) Pamidronate (Aredia) and zoledronate (Zometa) induced avascular necrosis of the jaws: a growing epidemic (Letter). J Oral Maxillofac Surg 61:1115
11. Ruggiero SL, Mehrotra B, Rosenberg TJ, Engroff S (2004) Osteonecrosis of the jaws associated with the use of bisphosphonates: a review of 63 cases. J Oral Maxillofac Surg 62:527
12. Migliorati CA, Schubert MM, Peterson DE, Seneda LM (2005) Bisphosphonate-associated osteonecrosis of mandibular and maxillary bone: an emerging oral complication of supportive cancer therapy. Cancer 104:83
13. Woo SB, Hellstein JW, Kalmar JR (2006) Systematic review: bisphosphonates and osteonecrosis of the jaws. Ann Intern Med 144:753
14. Nastro E, Musolino C, Allegra A, Oteri G et al (2007) Bisphosphonate-associated osteonecrosis of the jaw in patients with multiple myeloma and breast cancer. Acta Haematol 117(3):181–187
15. Ruggiero SL, Dodson TB, Assael LA, Landsberg R et al (2009) American Association of Oral and Maxillofacial Surgeons position paper on bisphosphonate-related osteonecrosis of the jaws-update. J Oral Maxillofac Surg 67(5 suppl.):2–12
16. Walter C, Al Nawas B, Grotz Ka, Thomas C et al (2008) Prevalence and risk factors of bisphosphonates osteonecrosis of the jaw in prostate cancer patients with advanced disease treated with zoledronate. Eur Urol 54(5):1066–1072
17. Ruggiero SL, Fantasia J, Carlson E (2006) Bisphosphonate-related osteonecrosis of the jaw: background and guidelines for diagnosis, staging and management. Oral Surge Oral Med Oral Pathol Oral Radiol Endod 102:433–441
18. Schwartz HC (2005) Osteonecrosis of the jaws: a complex group of disorders. J Oral Maxillofac Surg 63:1248–1249
19. Fantasia J (2009) Bisphosphonates—what the dentist needs to know: practical considerations. J Oral Maxillofac Surg 67(Suppl 1):53–60
20. Malden N, Beltes C, Lopes V (2009) Dental extractions and bisphosphonates: the assessment, consent and management, a proposed algorithm. Br Dent J 206(2):93–98

21. Bilezikian JP (2006) Osteonecrosis of the jaw —do bisphosphonates pose a risk? N Engl J Med 355:22
22. Assael LA (2009) Oral bisphosphonates as a cause of bisphosphonate related osteonecrosis of the jaws clinical findings assessment of risks and preventive strategies. J Oral Maxillofac Surg 67(11):35–43
23. Vahtsevanos K, Kyrgidis A, Verrou E et al (2009) Longitudinal cohort study of risk factors in cancer patients of bisphosphonate-related osteonecrosis of the jaw. J Clin Oncol 27(32): 5356–5362
24. Kyrgidis A (2009) Novel hypotheses in the etiopathogenesis of bisphosphonates related osteonecrosis of the jaws. J Oral Maxillofac Surg 67(11):2554
25. Hoff AO, Toth BB, Altundag K et al (2008) Frequency and risk factors associated with osteonecrosis of the jaw in cancer patients treated with intravenous bisphosphonates. J Bone Miner Res 23(6):826–836
26. Estilo CL, Van Poznak CH, Wiliams T et al (2008) Osteonecrosis of the maxilla and mandible in patients with advanced cancer treated with bisphosphonate therapy. Oncologist 13(8):911–920
27. Bisdas S, Chambron Pinho N, Smolarz A et al (2008) Bisphosphonate-induced osteonecrosis of the jaws CT and MRI spectrum of findings in 32 patients. Clin Radiol 63(1):71–77
28. Patschan D, Loddenkemper K, Buttgereit F (2001) Molecular mechanisms of glucocorticoid-induced osteoporosis. Bone 29:498–505
29. Meechan JG, Macgregor ID, Rogers SN et al (1988) The effect of smoking on immediate post-extraction socket fi lling with blood and on the incidence of painful socket. Br J Oral Maxillofac Surg 26:402–409
30. Sarasquete ME, Gonzáles M, San Miguel JF, Garcìa-Sanz R (2008) BRONJ is associated with polymorphisms of the cytochrome P450 CYP2C8 in multiple myeloma: a genome-wide single nucleotide analysis. Blood 111:2709
31. Migliorati CA, Casiglia J, Epstein J et al (2005) Managing the care of patients with bisphosphonate-associated osteonecrosis: an American Academy of Oral Medicine position paper. J Am Dent Assoc 136:1658–1668
32. Edwards BJ, Hellstein JW, Jacobsen PL et al (2006) Dental management of patients receiving oral bisphosphonate therapy: expert panel recommendations. J Am Dent Assoc 137: 1144–1150
33. Van den Wyngaert T, Huizing MT, Vermorken JB (2007) Osteonecrosis of the jaw related to the use of bisphosphonates. Curr Opin Oncol 19:315–322
34. Dimopoulos MA, Kastritis E, Bamia C et al (2009) Reduction of osteonecrosis of the jaw (ONJ) after implementation of preventive measures in patients with multiple myeloma treated with zoledronic acid. Ann Oncol 20(1):117–120
35. Ripamonti CI, Maniezzo M, Campa T et al (2009) Decreased occurrence of osteonecrosis of the jaw after implementation of dental preventive measures in solid tumour patients with bone metastasestreated with bisphosphonates The experience of the National Cancer Institute of Milan. Ann Oncol 20(1):137–145
36. Madrid C, Jaques B, Bouferrache K, Broome M (2007) Management of complications of bisphosphonates in oncology patients: jaw osteonecrosis. Rev Med Suisse 3(112): 1322–1324–6, 1329–31
37. Khosla S, Burr D, Cauley J et al (2007) Bisphosphonate-associated osteonecrosis of the jaw: report of a task force of the American Society for Bone and Mineral Research. J Bone Miner Res 22:1479
38. Lodi G, Sardella A, Salis A et al (2010) Tooth extraction in patients taking intravenous bisphosphonates: a preventive protocol and case series. J Oral Maxillofac Surg 68(1): 107–110
39. Saia G, Blandamura S, Bettini G, Tronchet A et al (2010) Occurrence of bisphosphonate-related osteonecrosis of the jaw after surgical tooth extraction. J Oral Maxillofac Surg 68(4):797–804

40. Marx RE, Cillo JE, Ulloa JJ (2007) Oral bisphosphonate-induced osteonecrosis: risk factors, prediction of risk using serum CTX testing, prevention, and treatment. J Oral Maxillofac Surg 65:2397
41. Montebugnoli L, Felicetti L, Gissi DB et al (2007) Bisphosphonate-associated osteonecrosis can be controlled by nonsurgical management. Oral Surg Oral Med Oral Pathol Oral Radiol Endod 104:473
42. Mavrokokki T, Cheng A, Stein B et al (2007) Nature and frequency of bisphosphonate-associated osteonecrosis of the jaws in Australia. J Oral Maxillofac Surg 65:415
43. Bell BM, Bell RE (2008) Oral bisphosphonates and dental implants: a retrospective study. J Oral Maxillofac Surg 66:1022
44. Black DM, Schwartz AV, Ensrud KE et al (2006) Effects of continuing or stopping alendronate after 5 years of treatment. The Fracture International Intervention Trial Long Term Extension (FLEX): a randomized trial. JAMA 296:2927
45. Grant BT, Amenedo C, Freeman K et al (2008) Outcomes of placing dental implants in patients taking oral bisphosphonates: a review of 115 cases. J Oral Maxillofac Surg 66:223
46. Bedogni A, Bettini G, Totola, et al. (2010) Oral bisphosphonate-associated osteonecrosis of the jaw after implant surgery: a case report and literature review. J Oral Maxillofac Surg 68:1662-1666
47. Rosen HN, Moses AC, Garber J et al (2000) Serum CTX: a new marker of bone resorption that shows treatment effect more often than other markers because of low coefficient of variability and large changes with bisphosphonates therapy. Calcif Tissue Int 66:100
48. Kwon YD, Kim DY, Ohe JY et al (2009) Correlation between serum C-terminal cross-linking telopeptide of type I collagen and staging of oral bisphosphonate-related osteonecrosis of the jaws. J Oral Maxillofac Surg 67(12):2644–2648
49. Lazarovici TS, Mesilaty-Gross S, Vered I et al (2010) Serologic bone markers for predicting development of osteonecrosis of the jaw in patients receiving bisphosphonates. J Oral Maxillofac Surg 68(9):2241–2247
50. Kunchur R, Need A, Hughes T, Goss A (2009) Clinical investigation of C-Terminal cross-linking telopeptide test in prevention ad management of bisphosphonate-associated osteonecrosis of the jaws. J Oral Maxillofac Surg 67(6):1167–1173
51. Schwartz H (2008) Serum CTX testing comment on J Oral. Maxillofac Surg 66(6): 1319–1320
52. Dodson TB (2010) Ctx and its role in managing patients exposed to oral bisphosphonates. J Oral Maxillofac Surg 68:487–494
53. Fleisher KE, Welch G, Kottal S et al (2010) Predicting risk for bisphosphonate-related osteonecrosis of the jaws: CTX versus radiographic markers. Oral Surg Oral Med Oral Pathol Oral Radiol Endod 110(4):509–516

Conservative Treatment: Oxygen-Ozone Therapy

11

Alessandro Agrillo

Abstract

Although surgery combined with antibiotic therapy forms the basis of most BIONJ treatment protocols, this approach is not always effective. Therefore, some authors have advocated bio-stimulation, such as achieved with oxygen-ozone therapy, to improve local repair mechanisms.

11.1 Introduction

One of the main features of bisphosphonates-induced osteonecrosis of the jaw (BIONJ) is the reduced vascularization of the bone tissue, with a consequent reduction in oxygen supply and cellular nutrition. Histologic studies have confirmed the continued presence of gaps arising from atrophy of the bone-tissue microvasculature, which explains the alternative name of this pathological entity, avascular osteonecrosis. Moreover, drug accumulation in the soft tissues lining the maxillary and mandibular skeletal structures augments the hypotrophic effect of bisphosphonates exposure.

Although surgery combined with antibiotic therapy forms the basis of most BIONJ treatment protocols, this approach is not always effective. Therefore, some authors have advocated bio-stimulation, such as achieved with oxygen-ozone therapy, to improve local repair mechanisms. Tissue hyperoxia has long been considered a useful therapeutic strategy for all lesions in which there is reduced tissue tropism. The benefits of this approach have been exploited, for example,

A. Agrillo (✉)
Maxillofacial Surgery Department,
University "La Sapienza" of Rome, Rome, Italy
e-mail: alessandro.agrillo@tiscali.it

F. S. De Ponte (ed.), *Bisphosphonates and Osteonecrosis of the Jaw: A Multidisciplinary Approach*, DOI: 10.1007/978-88-470-2083-2_11,

in the treatment of lesions arising from bacterial infection. While not yet recognized internationally, the addition of oxygen-ozone therapy to surgery and antibiotics has achieved encouraging results in patients with BIONJ.

11.2 Oxygen Therapy

Oxygen administered via a hyperbaric chamber (HBO) essentially uses capillary flow to reach the site of infection, where free radicals provided by macrophages together with natural-killer cells enhance the immune response. Oxygen also dissolves in the plasma and thus reaches the tissues [1]. Thus, HBO as well as ozone therapy creates adverse conditions for anaerobic bacteria and improves the growth of healthy tissue, increasing the peripheral O_2 concentration. Furthermore the release of free radicals reduces or inhibits bacterial DNA replication, especially in hypoxic or hypotrophic tissues.

The use of HBO in BIONJ has been studied by several investigators. The reactive oxygen and nitrogen atoms produced in response to HBO positively modulate the intracellular redox-sensitive molecular signals involved in bone turnover. Currently, randomized trials are aimed at establishing the relationship between HBO and the activity of osteoclasts, in order to determine the physiological basis of the encouraging clinical results obtained with oxygen therapy [2].

11.3 Ozone Therapy

Ozone (O_3) is made up of three oxygen atoms and has a characteristic garlic-like smell (the same as sometimes accompanies rain just released from the clouds). Its chemical structure is a resonance hybrid of three possible configurations, making it a highly reactive molecule. In the gaseous form at 20°C, ozone has a half-life of 3 days, but in aqueous solution its half-life is only 20 min; in the liquid state it is explosive. Therefore ozone cannot be preserved and must be produced as needed. The healing power of ozone, either alone or in combination with other therapeutic agents, in different diseases is well established. Its most important features are: (a) its antimicrobial activity against aerobic and anaerobic bacteria (especially *Staphylococcus aureus*), fungi, and viruses; (b) its stimulation of the circulatory system, increasing the synthesis of hemoglobin and the production of red blood cells, thus promoting tissue oxygenation; (c) as a modulator of immune cells, acting as a cytokine and increasing phagocytosis and diapedesis by phagocytes; (d) as a stimulator of angiogenesis as well as fibroblasts; and (e) its ability to reduce pain [3–8].

Ozone therapy is administered by a variety of methods according to clinical needs. Systemically, ozonated autohemotherapy consists of exposure to an oxygen-ozone gas mixture [9], such as in the treatment of the vasculature of the lower limbs in patients with chronic atherosclerosis, ischemic heart disease, or age-related macular degeneration [6]. Intramuscular injections are currently

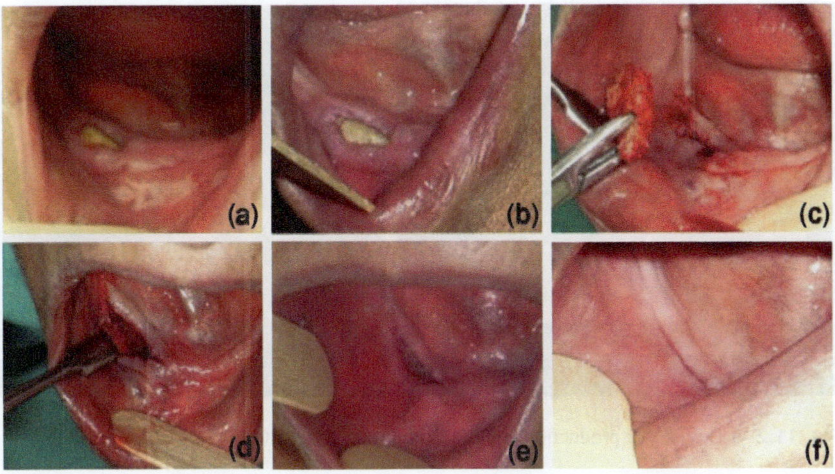

Fig. 11.1 Osteonecrotic lesion. **a** Osteonecrotic lesion in a patient with multiple myeloma. **b** Lesion after one cycle of ozone therapy. **c, d** Sequestrectomy. **e, f** Covering of the mandibular crest after 1 week and after 1 month

widely used for the treatment of chronic arthritis or herniated discs. Other methods are insufflation, ozonated water, and ozonated oil [10].

In a 1999 study, Steinhart used a rabbit model to evaluate the use of localized ozone in association with antibiotic therapy and surgery in the treatment of refractory osteomyelitis of the head and neck. The resulting positive effects were ascribed not only to the activation of fibroblasts and angiogenesis, but also to ozone's bactericidal actions, especially against anaerobes and *S. aureus*. Moreover, in this form of treatment many of the negative systemic effects of other commonly used reagents could be eliminated [11].

The use of ozone in the treatment of BIONJ was first reported in the literature in 2006 [12]. Those authors introduced ozone therapy as a support to surgery and antibiotics, reporting an improvement of BIONJ-related symptoms in 90% of the cases. While it soon became apparent that ozone therapy could not replace existing therapies, it can be considered as an essential supplement to pre-and post-surgical treatment, improving patients' quality of life [12].

In later studies on larger groups of patients, ozone's effects on angiogenesis and the immune system were found to include the formation of areas of bone sequestrum and an increase in the vascularity of the bone underlying the lesion, resulting in the formation of granulating tissue from the mucosa. The removal of the sequestrum then exposes an area below the regeneration process, which often does not need additional surgery for closure [13, 14] (Fig. 11.1). However, if the surgical procedure consists of deep ablation of the bone lesion, in the search for vascularized tissue, this is not always achievable. The adoption of different modes of ozone administration, such as auto-hemotransfusion or the administration of ozonized water, could, in the near future, increase the success rate in the treatment of this difficult disease.

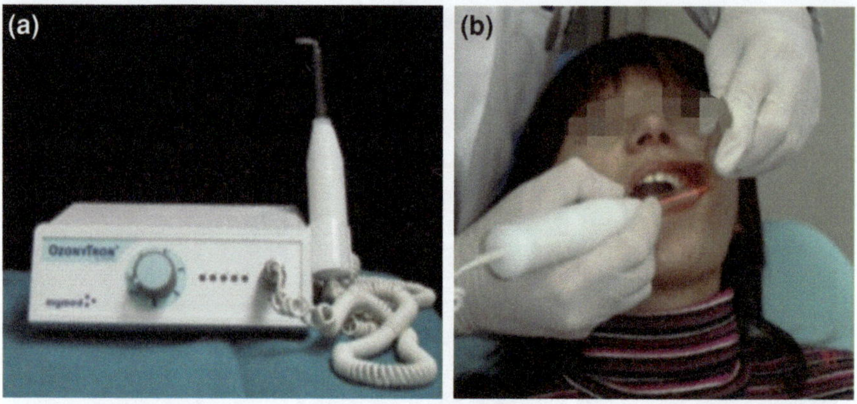

Fig. 11.2 **a** Device for production and application of gaseous O_3. **b** Application technique

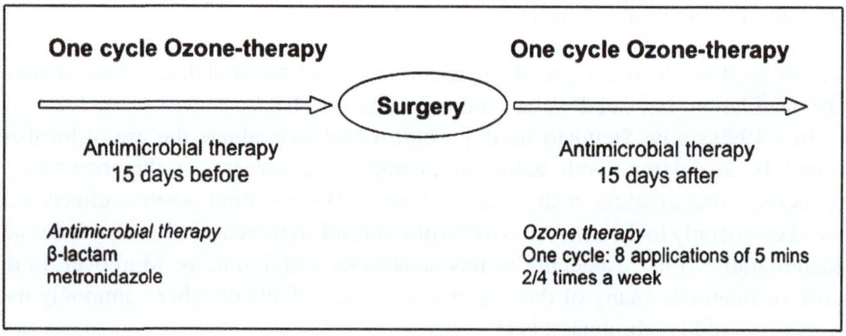

Fig. 11.3 Therapeutic protocol with ozone therapy, antimicrobial therapy and non invasive surgical treatment

11.3.1 Ozone Protocol

Current protocols consist of minimally invasive surgery combined with cycles of topical ozone therapy before and afterwards, using a device such as the Ozonitron, which administers ozone by topical insufflations (Fig. 11.2). Each cycle corresponds to eight 3-min sessions at a frequency of 2–4 sessions per week. In addition, all patients undergo antibiotic therapy with β-lactam antibiotics such as metronidazole [14] (Fig. 11.3).

Surgical treatment involves bony curettage of the lesion, preferably performed without the use of a drill to minimize trauma, or sequestrectomy. In almost all cases, mucosal flaps are not created during surgery nor are sutures used. Instead, simple packing of the residual cavity with lubricated gauzes is usually adequate. Following treatment, patients should be given an oral hygiene protocol, including rinses with sodium hypochlorite 0.05%.

References

1. Coppola L, Verrazzo G (1992) Oxygen-ozone therapy and haemorheological parameters in peripheral chronic arterial disease. Trombosi e Aterosclerosi 3(2): marzo-aprile
2. Freiberger JJ (2009) The utility of hyperbaric oxygen in the treatment of biphosphonate-related osteonecrosis of the jaws. J Oral Maxillofac Surg 67:30
3. Dayas A, Boughton BJ, Das BC (1983) Ozone killing action against bacterial and fungal species microbiological testing of a domestic ozone generator. J Clin Pathol 36:1102–1104
4. Bocci V (1996) Ozone as bioregulator: Pharmacology and toxicology of ozone-therapy today. J Biol Regul Homeost Agents 10:31–53
5. Bocci V, Paulesu L (1990) Studies on the biological effects of ozone: 1. Induction of interferon gamma on humen leucocytes. Haematologica 75:510–515
6. Bocci V (2004) Ozone as Janus. Mediators of Inflammation 13(1):3–11
7. Muller P, Guggenheim B, Shmidlin P (2007) Efficacy of gasiform ozone and photodynamic therapy on a multispecies oral biofilm in vitro. Eur J Oral Sci 115:77–80
8. Azarpazhooh A, Limeback H (2008) The application of ozone in dentistry: a systematic review of literature. J Dentist 36:104–116
9. Wolff HH (1974) Die Behandlung peripherer Durchblutungsstőrungen mit Ozon. Erfahrungsheilkunde 23:181–184
10. Morrey BF, Dunn JM, Helmbach RD, Davis J (1979) Hyperbaric oxygen and chronic osteomyelitis. Clin Orthop 144:121–127
11. Steinhart H, Shulz S, Mutters R (1999) Evaluation of ozonated oxygen in an experimental animal model of osteomyelitis as a further treatment option for skull base osteomyelitis. Eur Arch Othorhinolaringol 256:153–157
12. Agrillo A, Petrucci MT, Tedaldi M, Mustazza MC, Marino SM, Gallucci C, Iannetti G (2006) New therapeutic protocol in the treatment of avascular necrosis of the jaws. J Craniofacial Surg 17(6):1080–1083
13. Agrillo A, Ungari C, Filiaci F, Priore P, Iannetti G (2007) Ozone therapy in the treatment of avascular bisphosphonate-related jaw osteonecrosis. J Craniofac Surg 18(5):1071–1075
14. Agrillo A, Sassano P, Rinna C, Priore P, Iannetti G (2007) Ozone therapy in extractive surgery on patients treated with bisphosphonates. J Craniofac Surg 18(5):1068–1070

Conservative Treatment: LASER (Biostimulation and Minimally Invasive Surgical Treatment)

12

Paolo Vescovi

Abstract

Several studies have shown a positive effect of low-level laser therapy (LLLT) using different wavelengths (argon, CO_2, He-neon, Er:YAG, diode, Nd:YAG, and KTP) on the healing process in a wide range of cutaneous, mucosal, and bone disorders. LLLT reportedly stimulates osteoclast activity to promote bone resorption and remodeling. Soft-tissue healing is also improved by LLLT. The transformation of fibroblasts into myofibroblasts can accelerate the healing of skin and mucosa. In particular, in conditions characterized by avascular necrosis, such as bisphosphonates-induced osteonecrosis of the jaw (BIONJ), it is essential to stimulate vascularization and soft-tissue tropism through an increase in blood flow by means of angiogenesis, capillary growth, and an increase in growth factor release. Laser can be used in the conservative surgical treatment of BIONJ patients. The procedure involves the vaporization of necrotic bone until healthy bone is reached. The minimal penetration of the erbium laser (0.1 mm) guarantees safety and allows for precise, minimally invasive surgery, inducing a much lower increase in bone temperature than conventional rotary tools (cold ablation). One undoubted advantage of this technique for BIONJ patients is the bactericidal action of the laser beam, in particular versus Actinomyces and anaerobes species. These considerations support the effectiveness of LLLT in the treatment of jawbone and mucosal defects related to BIONJ development or following tooth extractions in patients under bisphosphonates therapy. Thus, minimally invasive laser-assisted surgical treatment appears to be a promising approach for BIONJ management.

P. Vescovi (✉)
Sezione di Odontostomatologia, Azienda Ospedaliero-Universitaria di Parma, Parma, Italy
e-mail: paolo.vescovi@unipr.it

F. S. De Ponte (ed.), *Bisphosphonates and Osteonecrosis of the Jaw: A Multidisciplinary Approach*, DOI: 10.1007/978-88-470-2083-2_12,

12.1 Introduction

Current forms of therapy for bisphosphonates-induced osteonecrosis of the jaw (BIONJ) are controversial and their use remains problematic. Moreover, there are no evidence-based guidelines on the management BIONJ and no prospective studies reporting good results during long term follow-up. Patients experience an improvement in symptoms following the use of oral antimicrobial rinses in combination with oral systemic antibiotic therapy. However, they often require a combination of antibiotic therapy, long-term maintenance, or a course of intravenous antibiotic therapy. The objective of each treatment is to alleviate pain, reduce infection, and stabilize progression of the disease. Different minimally invasive strategies of BIONJ management, such as biostimulative laser therapy and laser surgery, have been described in the last five years.

12.2 Low Level Laser Therapy

Avascular necrotic bone, bacterial and fungal colonies, and abundant inflammatory infiltration are frequently observed in BIONJ [1]. Amino-bisphosphonates (N-BPs) inhibit turnover and the repair capacity of the bone after microdamages [2, 3]. In addition, these drugs decrease epithelial cell proliferation via the reduction of farnesyl diphosphate synthetase and exhibit anti-angiogenic properties, including the inhibition of vascular endothelial growth factor (VEGF) production [4, 5]. The alteration of angiogenesis may have important effects on both the quality and the quantity of bone vascularization, possibly altering the response to trauma and infections [6].

Several studies have shown the positive effects of low-level laser therapy (LLLT) with different wavelengths on the healing process in a wide range of cutaneous, mucosal, and bone disorders. These observations support the possible validity of laser biostimulation in the treatment of BIONJ [7]. As reported in the literature, the laser wavelengths with biostimulant effects in the maxillofacial area are: argon, CO_2, He-neon, Er:YAG, diode, Nd:YAG, and KTP [8].

The laser beam produces several changes in cellular metabolism. Particularly, light is absorbed by the primary photo-acceptors, which triggers the usual cell regulatory "machinery." The intensity of the effects is based on the cells' physiological state during irradiation and on the applied wavelength. The efficacy of LLLT probably involves a photochemical mechanism, with photo-energy being firstly absorbed by intracellular mitochondrial chromophores and then converted to metabolic energy, thereby involving the respiratory cytochrome chain [9–12]. Laser light causes a build-up of singlet oxygen, which acts as a free radical and thus alters the production of ATP and the formation of transmembrane electrochemical proton gradients in mitochondria. The irradiation seems to increase the release of prostaglandin E2 (PGE2), contributing to bone and mucosal healing [13]. A two-step mechanism is involved in the interaction between irradiation and bone repair: (1) osteoblast activation to produce bone matrix and (2) an inhibitory photobiological mechanism that results in decreased osteoblast activity. In addition, LLLT has been reported to stimulate osteoclast activity to promote bone resorption and remodeling [14]. Stimulatory effects on bone formation have been obtained by repeated irradiation with a low energy dose for a given period of time rather than by unique irradiation at the same total energy dose.

Soft-tissue healing is also improved by LLLT. In particular, there is a shortening of the exudation phase and a stimulation of repair processes, thus promoting the formation of granulation tissue. The transformation of fibroblasts into myofibroblasts can accelerate the healing of skin and mucosa [15]. This is of particular relevance in avascular necrosis conditions, such as BIONJ, where it is very important to stimulate vascularization and soft-tissue tropism.

Many authors have reported an LLLT-mediated increase in blood flow by means of angiogenesis and capillary growth as well as an increase in growth factor release (TGF, PDGF, bFGF, IL6, IL8, IL1α). More rapid formation of collagen type I and III and an increase in collagen deposition have also been reported in many experiments, both in vitro and in vivo [16, 17].

A significant effect of laser irradiation is the antibacterial activity shown in in vitro studies and animal models. This is of relevance in BIONJ since biofilms have been identified on the bone/tooth/mucosal surfaces around the necrotic lesions and were found to contain *Actinomyces* spp, *Eikinella*, *Peptostreptococcus*, and *Legionella*. However, it is unclear whether infection is a primary or secondary event in BIONJ pathophysiology [18]. The effectiveness of laser treatment depends on the wavelength used, and thus on the energy delivered, and the bacterial species being irradiated. Nonetheless, the exact mechanism by which laser irradiation exerts its bactericidal effect has not yet been determined, but it likely involves photochemical or photothermal effects [19]. The efficacy of the bactericidal effect of Nd:YAG and diode lasers has been demonstrated in endodontic and periodontal therapy, in which the laser beam caused a decrease in the number of bacteria in different models: infected extracted teeth, capillary tubes, and microplate [20–22].

On the basis of our experience, BIONJ patients were treated with Nd:YAG laser biostimulation and antibiotic therapy (2 g amoxicillin and 1.5 g metronidazole per day for 2 weeks). The Nd:YAG laser (wavelength 1,064 nm, power 1.25 W, frequency 15 Hz, fiber 320-μm diameter) used to administer LLLT was defocused at a distance of 1–2 mm from the tissue for 1 min (PD 1,865 W/cm^2, fluence per pulse 124.33 J/cm^2, cumulative fluence 746 J/cm^2) for five consecutive applications. Patients received laser applications twice a week for an average period of 1 month. Clinical success with improvement in symptoms was obtained in 60% of the patients with a minimum follow-up of 6 months. In patients treated with medical therapy only, no site showed a transition to stage 0 (complete mucosal healing) in contrast to patients treated with medical therapy combined with LLLT, which resulted in 41% of the lesions showing a transition to stage 0 in patients with a mean follow-up of 7.5 months (range 3–18 months) [23].

Other authors observed an important reduction of pain, edema, size of bone exposure, pus, fistulas, and halitosis in BIONJ patients after 4 weeks of treatment with LLLT, administered with diode laser [24, 25].

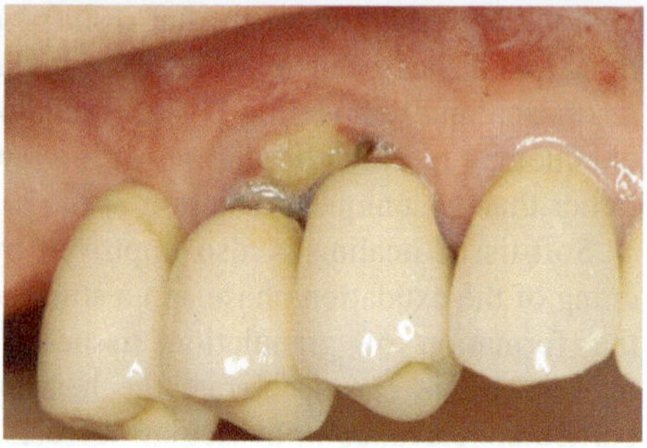

Fig. 12.1 Clinical features of stage I BIONJ in areas in the proximity of dental implants. This 64-year-old woman with osteoporosis had been treated with alendronate for 9 years

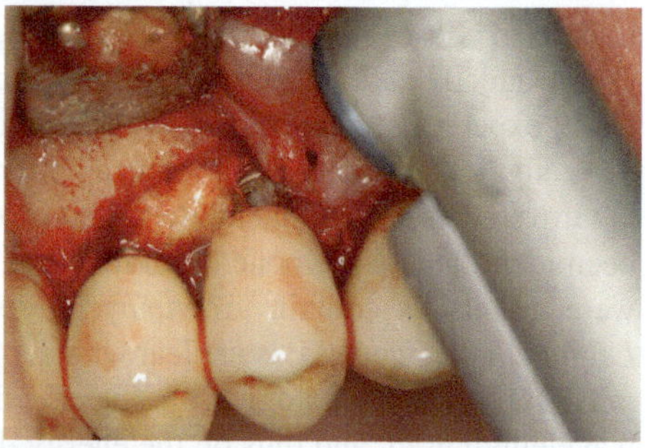

Fig. 12.2 Vaporization of necrotic bone using an Er:YAG laser (non-contact mode)

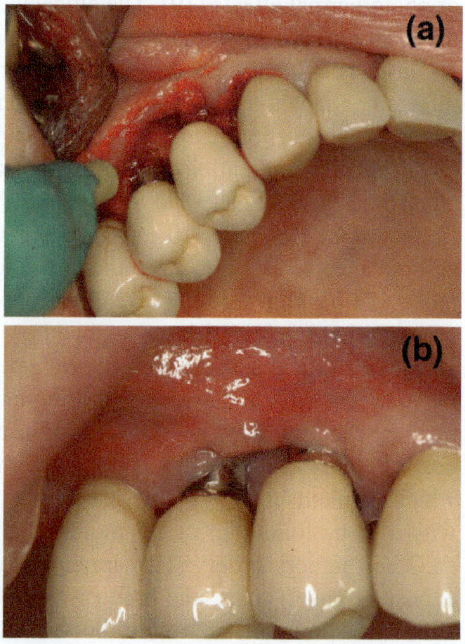

Fig. 12.3 **a** Biostimulation of the surgical area using low-level laser therapy (Nd:Yag laser). **b** At 3-weeks follow-up, there is complete clinical healing

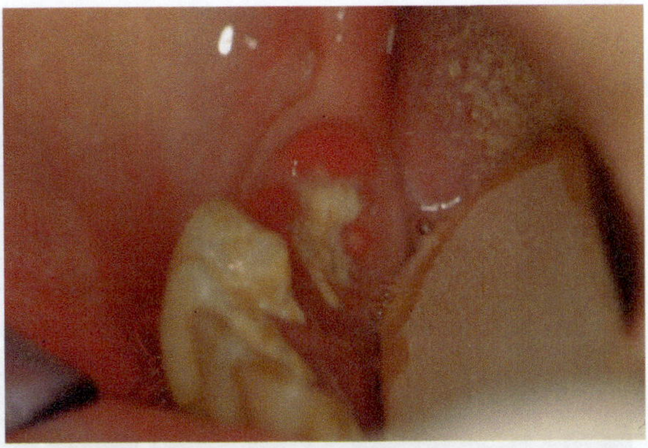

Fig. 12.4 Stage I BIONJ of the lower jaw in an area of chronic trauma associated with complete denture wearing. This 67-year-old woman with breast cancer and bone metastases had been treated with zoledronate for 8 months

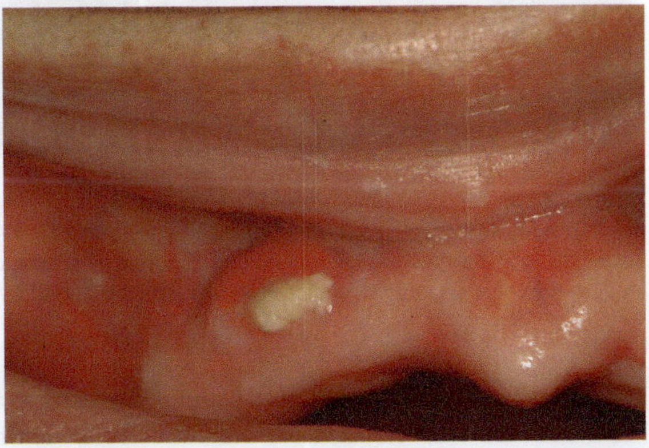

Fig. 12.5 Stage I BIONJ of the maxilla in the same patient as in Fig. 12.4

LLLT performed with different wavelengths appears to be a significant modality of treatment for BIONJ. As a safe, non-invasive procedure that is well tolerated and without side effects, it is recommended for both cancer and non-cancer patients and can be of great help in cases of BIONJ that require non-surgical management.

12.3 Minimally Invasive Laser Surgery

The non-invasive management of BIONJ is related to preventing the possible extension of the necrotic process. However, until recently, scientific reports in the literature stated that in stage I and II disease better results can be obtained with early surgical therapy than with medical treatment only [26–28].

Many authors have reported clinical success with traditional conservative surgical treatment (soft sequestrectomy and debridement) accompanied by antibiotic therapy and local chlorhexidine rinses, with complete mucosal closure in 53–78% of patients [29, 30].

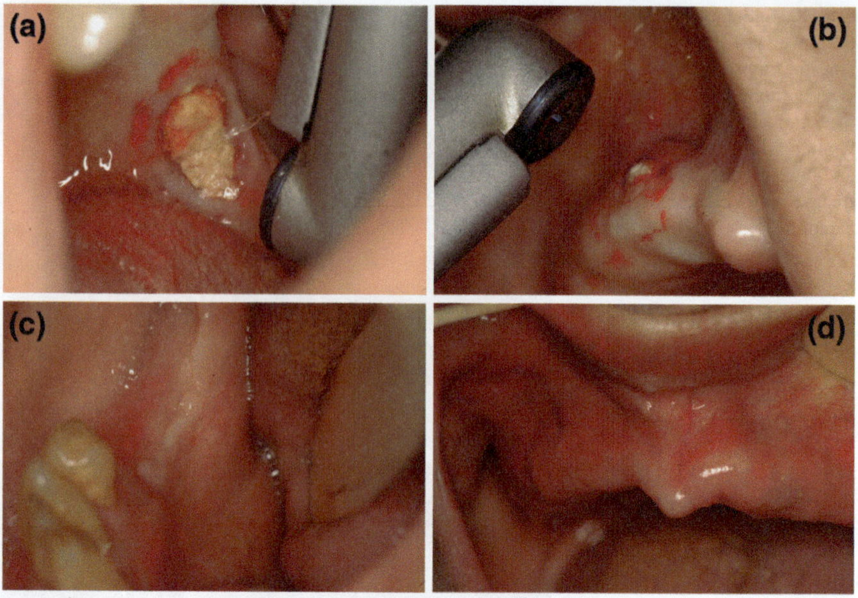

Fig. 12.6 **a** Vaporization of mandibular necrotic bone through Er:YAG laser (non-contact mode). **b** Vaporization of maxillary necrotic bone using Er:YAG laser. **c** At 1-month follow-up, there is complete mucosal healing of the mandibular treated site in shown in (**a**). **d** At 1-month follow-up, there is complete mucosal healing of the maxillary treated site shown in (**b**)

Laser can be used in BIONJ patients for conservative surgery. The procedure involves the vaporization of necrotic bone until healthy bone is reached. An Er:YAG solid-state laser is used, in which the active medium is a crystal of yttrium-aluminium-garnet doped with erbium. The radiation wavelength of 2.94 μm produces excellent absorption of hydroxyapatite and water. The erbium laser penetrates only very slightly (0.1 mm), guaranteeing the safety of the procedure and allowing for precise, minimally invasive treatment. Moreover, a much lower increase in bone temperature is induced than is the case with conventional rotary tools (cold ablation) (Figs. 12.1, 12.2, 12.3, 12.4, 12.5, 12.6). As noted above, one undoubted advantage of this technique for BIONJ treatment is the bactericidal action of the laser beam against *Actinomyces* and anaerobic species. Many authors reported quicker healing of the bone and of the coating tissues following erbium laser surgery [31]. Histological examination of the laser-treated bone has shown improved tissue repair compared to bone treated with conventional tools [32, 33].

An evaluation of the peripheral bone damage induced by the different cutting systems demonstrated that all sections obtained with Er:YAG laser were better than those obtained by piezosurgery, high-speed drill, and low-speed drill. Er:YAG laser resulted in poor peripheral carbonization with a regular incision without a residual bone smear layer [34]. The erbium laser technique enables

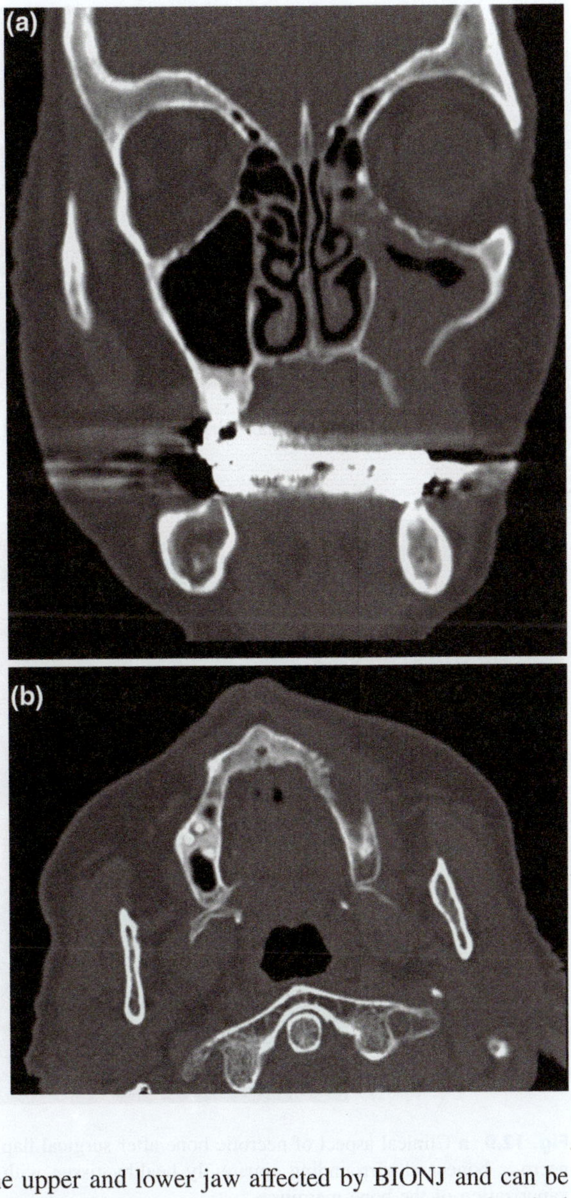

Fig. 12.7 **a** Computed tomography scan of the maxillofacial region, with radiographic evidence of involvement of the left maxillary sinus (stage III BIONJ) in a 72-year-old woman with osteoporosis and rheumatoid arthritis who had been treated with corticosteroids and alendronate for 10 years. **b** Computed tomography scan of the maxillofacial region, with radiographic evidence of bone necrosis in the patient described in (**a**)

resection of the bones of the upper and lower jaw affected by BIONJ and can be performed using local anesthesia (Figs. 12.7, 12.8, 12.9, 12.10). Surgical debridement is also possible, with gradual evaporation of the necrotic bone at depths increasingly close to healthy bone. The minimally invasive technique of evaporation allows the sectioned bone surfaces to be made regular and the creation of micro-perforations at the base for renewed vascularization [35]. In our experience, BIONJ sites were treated with Er:YAG laser at very short pulses (VSP mode: pulse duration of 100 μs) and at a setting of 300 mJ, 30 Hz and 60 J/cm^2 of

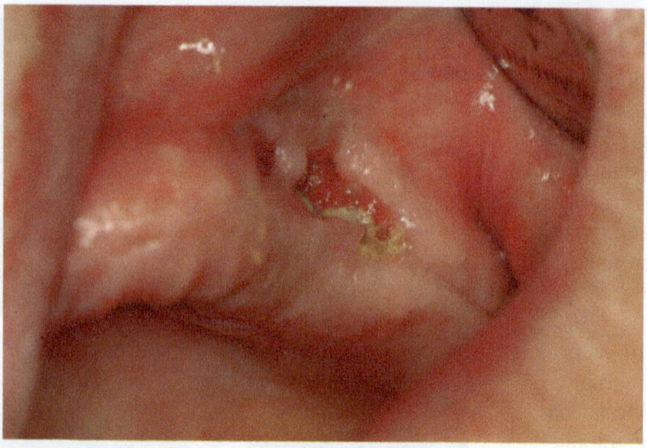

Fig. 12.8 Clinical features of maxillary BIONJ (same patient as in Fig. 12.7)

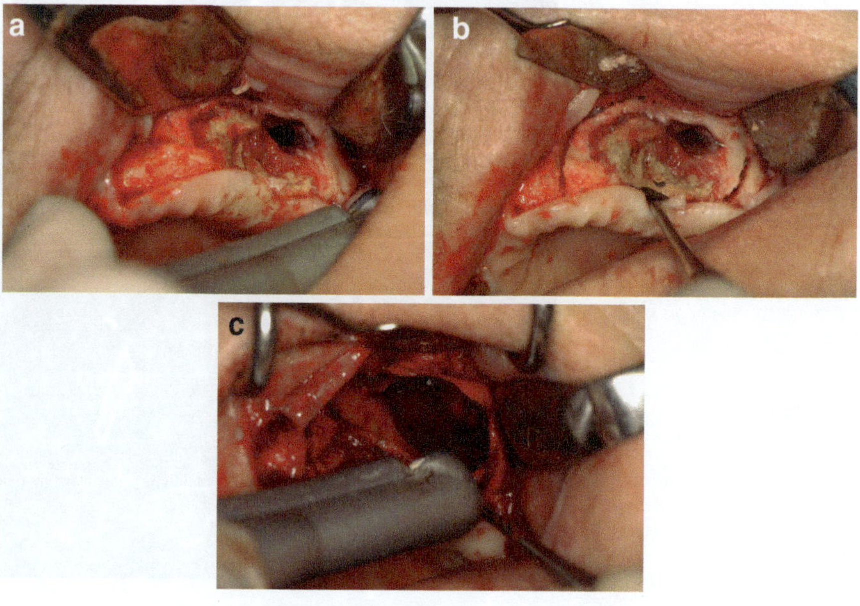

Fig. 12.9 **a** Clinical aspect of necrotic bone after surgical flap opening. **b** Surgical resection of necrotic bone and surrounding apparently healthy tissue with Er:YAG laser. **c** Er:YAG laser vaporization of the bone margins

fluence; the laser device was used in non-contact or near-contact mode. Clinical success was obtained in cancer and non-cancer patients for 97% of BIONJ sites, with a complete mucosal healing in 90% of the cases for an average period of 13 months of follow up [36, 37]. Other authors reported similar results with laser surgery [38, 39].

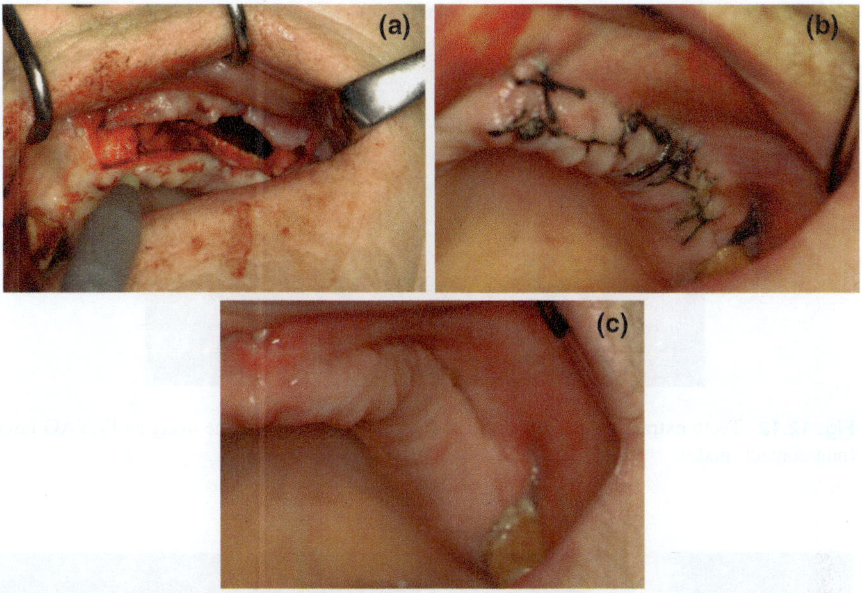

Fig. 12.10 **a** Biostimulation of the surgical area using low-level laser therapy (Nd:Yag laser). **b** At 1-week follow-up. **c** At 1-month follow-up, there is complete mucosal healing

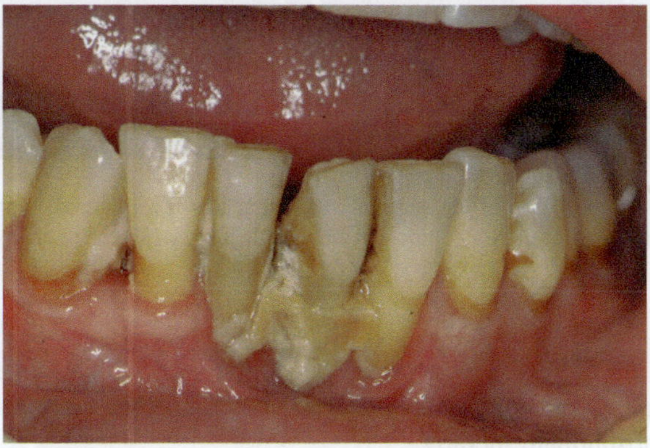

Fig. 12.11 Clinical features of stage II BIONJ in a 66-year-old periodontopathic patient with multiple myeloma who had been treated with zoledronate for 9 months

12.4 Laser and Preventive Measures

Many expert panels have developed various documents on preventive strategies. These documents are aimed at specialists involved in the multidisciplinary management of BIONJ patients. Dental surgical procedures (tooth extractions,

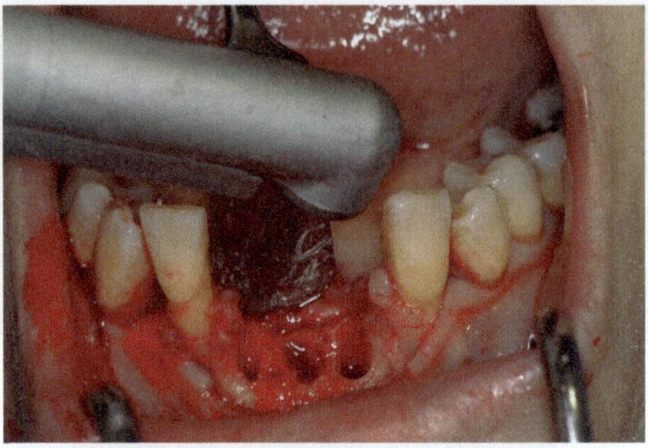

Fig. 12.12 Teeth extraction, vaporization, and decontamination of bone using an Er:YAG laser (non-contact mode)

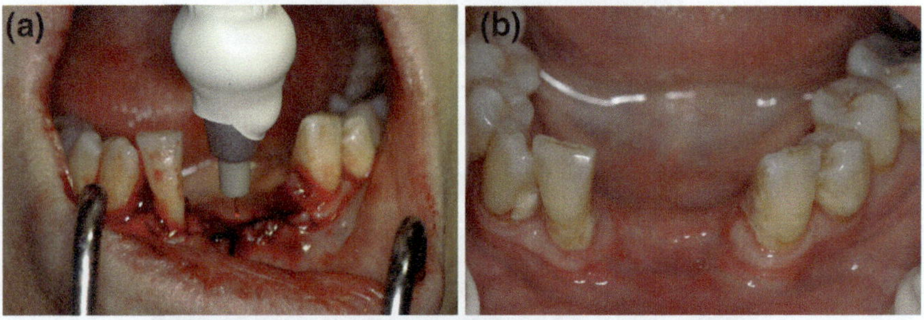

Fig. 12.13 **a** Biostimulation of the surgical area using low-level laser therapy (Nd:Yag laser). **b** At 2-months follow-up, there is complete mucosal healing of the site shown in (**a**)

bone remodeling of severe exostoses, endodontic surgery) and urgent periodontal treatment (scaling and root planing) should be completed before the commencement of bisphosphonate therapy.

Surgical trauma is a recognized predisposing factor to BIONJ development, although there are also significant percentages of spontaneous forms, as reported in the literature [40]. Tooth extractions and oral surgical interventions should thus be avoided (unless urgently necessary) because they increase the risk of BIONJ, by about eight-fold in both cancer and non-cancer patients [41] When a surgical procedure becomes unavoidable, antibiotic treatment with amoxicillin (2 g/day) 3 days prior to and 2 weeks after the intervention must be prescribed [42]. Laser treatment for bactericidal as well as biostimulatory effects can improve the outcome of dental invasive procedures by inducing bone and mucosal healing (Figs. 12.11, 12.12, 12.13) [43, 44].

12.5 Conclusions

Despite the many reports in the literature, optimal BIONJ therapy remains an unresolved issue and there are no evidence-based guidelines. The current discussion revolves around two opposite approaches: invasive versus non-invasive treatment. Regardless of the chosen strategy, the main objectives of treatment are to alleviate pain, reduce infection, stabilize disease progression, and, of course, obtain closure of the exposed bone.

Antibiotic therapy represents a non-invasive, valid solution to manage the symptoms of BIONJ, but the long-term results regarding complete mucosal healing are worse than those obtained through a surgical approach. However, the elderly or cancer patients may be debilitated by their malignancy, chemotherapy, or comorbidities and thus unable to tolerate the side effects of prolonged therapeutic antibiotic schedules. In these cases, LLLT (associated with medical therapy) may be more beneficial in the treatment of BIONJ lesions, especially when surgery is not an option. The diffuse forms of BIONJ require extensive bone resection after a careful evaluation of the patient's general conditions, including disease evolution, age, performance status, and life expectancy. However, a review of the literature showed less satisfactory results for stage III lesions than for lower stages. Based on this result, patients with minimal bone exposure should be considered as candidates for conservative surgical strategies.

In addition, in general, the status and life expectancy of cancer patients must always to be considered in the decision to perform extensive surgery. One of the exclusion criteria is the contraindication of surgery under general anesthesia. This places important limits on the surgical procedure and confirms the choice for early minimally invasive laser-assisted surgical therapy in patients with stage I and stage II BIONJ.

Erbium laser permits bone resection or surgical debridement even when the procedure is performed under local anesthesia. The necrotic bone is gradually vaporized, until healthy bone is reached. The minimally invasive technique of evaporation allows the sectioned bone surfaces to be made regular. Furthermore, it can be used to create micro-perforations at the base for renewed vascularization. Additional advantages of laser therapy are the bactericidal and biostimulatory action of the laser beam, resulting in better post-operative recovery. Taken together, these considerations support the effectiveness of LLLT in the treatment of jawbone and mucosal defects related to BIONJ development or following tooth extractions in patients under bisphosphonate therapy. Thus, minimally invasive laser-assisted surgical treatment appears to be a promising approach for BIONJ management.

References

1. Sonis ST, Watkins BA, Lyng GD, Lerman MA, Anderson KC (2009) Bony changes in the jaws of rats treated with zoledronic acid and dexamethasone before dental extractions mimic bisphosphonate-related osteonecrosis in cancer patients. Oral Oncol 45:164–172

2. Fleisch H (1998) Bisphosphonates: mechanisms of action. Endocr Rev 19:80–100
3. Sarin J, DeRossi SS, Akintoye SO (2008) Updates on bisphosphonates and potential pathobiology of bisphosphonate-induced jaw osteonecrosis. Oral Dis 14:277–285
4. Reid IR, Bolland MJ, Grey AB (2007) Is bisphosphonate-associated osteonecrosis of the jaw caused by soft tissue toxicity? Bone 41:318–320
5. Landesberg R, Cozin M, Cremers S et al (2008) Inhibition of oral mucosal cell wound healing by bisphosphonates. J Oral Maxillofac Surg 66:839–847
6. Green JR (2004) Bisphosphonates: preclinical review. Oncologist 9:3–13
7. Vescovi P, Merigo E, Meleti M, Manfredi M (2006) Bisphosphonate-associated osteonecrosis (BON) of the jaws: a possible treatment? J Oral Maxillofac Surg 64:1460–1462
8. Gutknecht N (2007) Proceedings of the 1st international workshop of evidence-based dentistry on laser in dentistry. Quintessence Publishing, Chicago
9. Khadra M, Kasem N, Haanaes HR, Ellingsen JE, Lyngstadaas SP (2004) Enhancement of bone formation in rat calvarial bone defects using low-level laser therapy. Oral Surg Oral Med Oral Pathol Oral Radiol Endod 97:693–700
10. Bradley P, Tunér J (2007) Laser phototherapy in dentistry. In: Proceedings of the 1st international workshop of evidence-based dentistry on laser in dentistry. Quintessence Publishing, Chicago
11. Bjordal JM, Couppé C, Chow RT, Tunér J, Ljunggren EA (2003) A systematic review of low level laser therapy with location-specific doses for pain from chronic disorders. Aust J Physiother 49:107–116
12. Bjordal JM (2005) Can a Cochrane review in controversial areas be biased? A sensitivity analysis based on the protocol of a systematic Cochrane review low level laser therapy in osteoarthritis. Photomed Laser Surg 23:453–458
13. Garavello-Freitas I, Baranauskas V, Joazeiro PP et al (2003) Low-power laser irradiation improves histomorphometrical parameters and bone matrix organization during tibia wound healing in rats. J Photochem Photobiol B 70:81–89
14. Medrado AR, Pugliese LS, Reis SR, Andrade ZA (2003) Influence of low level laser therapy on wound healing and its biological action upon myofibroblasts. Lasers Surg Med 32:239–244
15. Bayat M, Vasheghani MM, Razavi N (2006) Effect of low-level helium-neon laser therapy on the healing of third-degree burns in rats. J Photochem Photobiol B 83:87–93
16. Pessoa ES, Melhado RM, Theodoro LH, Garcia VG (2004) A histologic assessment of the influence of low-intensity laser therapy on wound healing in steroid-treated animals. Photomed Laser Surg 22:199–204
17. Rabelo SB, Villaverde AB, Nicolau R, Salgado MC, Melo Mda S, Pacheco MT (2006) Comparison between wound healing in induced diabetic and nondiabetic rats after low-level laser therapy. Photomed Laser Surg 24:474–479
18. Sedghizadeh PP, Kumar SK, Gorur A, Schaudinn C, Shuler CF, Costerton JW (2008) Identification of microbial biofilms in osteonecrosis of the jaws secondary to bisphosphonate therapy. J Oral Maxillofac Surg 66:767–775
19. Rocca J-P (2008) Les lasers en odontologie. Editions CdP—Wolters Kluver France—Avril
20. Gutknecht N, Raoufi P, Frenzen R, Lampert F (2002) Reduction of specific microorganism in periodontal pockets with the aim of an Nd:YAG laser. An in vivo study. J Oral Laser Appl 2:175–180
21. Folwaczny M, Mehl A, Jordan C, Hickel R (2002) Antibacterial effects of pulsed Nd:YAG laser radiation at different energy settings in root canals. J Endod 1:24–29
22. Vescovi P, Merigo E, Conti S et al (2010) Bactericidal effect on Nd:YAG laser on *Staphylococcus aureus* and *Actinomyces israelii*: preliminary results. Lasers Med Sci 25:S42
23. Vescovi P, Merigo E, Manfredi M, Meleti M, Fornaini M, Bonanini M, Rocca JP, Nammour S (2008) Nd:YAG laser biostimulation in the treatment of bisphosphonate-associated necrosis of the jaw: clinical experience in 28 cases. Photomed Laser Surg 26:37–46
24. Scoletta M, Arduino PG, Reggio L, Delmasso P, Mozzati M (2010) Effect of low-level laser irradiation on bisphosphonate-induced osteonecrosis of the jaws: preliminary results of prospective study. Photomed Laser Surg 110:46–53

25. Romeo U, Galanakis A, Marias C, Vecchio AD, Tenore G, Palaia G, Vescovi P, Polimeni A (2011) Observation of pain control in patients with bisphosphonate-induced osteonecrosis using low level laser therapy: preliminary results. Photomed Laser Surg 29(7):447–452. doi:10.1089/pho.2010.2835. Epub 16 Jan 2011
26. Vescovi P, Merigo E, Meleti M, Manfredi M (2008) Early surgical approach preferable to medical therapy for bisphosphonate-related osteonecrosis of the jaw. J Oral Maxillofac Surg 66:931–933
27. Wutzl A, Biedermann E, Wanschitz F et al (2008) Treatment results of bisphosphonate-related osteonecrosis of the jaws. Head Neck 30:1224–1230
28. Markose G, Mackenzie FR, Currie WJ, Hislop WS (2009) Bisphosphonate osteonecrosis: a protocol for surgical management. Br J Oral Maxillofac Surg 47:294–297
29. Van den Wyngaert T, Claeys T, Huizing MT, Vermorken JB, Fossion E (2009) Initial experience with conservative treatment in cancer patients with osteonecrosis of the jaws (ONJ) and predictor outcomes. Ann Oncol 2:331–336
30. Stockmann P, Vairaktaris E, Wehrhan F et al (2010) Osteotomy and primary wound closure in bisphosphonate-associated osteonecrosis of the jaw: a prospective clinical study with 12 months follow-up. Support Care Cancer 18:449–460
31. Vescovi P, Romeo U, Merigo E et al (2011) Use of laser therapy in the treatment of jaw bone diseases. Dent Cadmos 79:133–148
32. Pourzarandian A, Watanabe H, Aoki A et al (2004) Histological and TEM examination of early stages of bone healing after Er:YAG laser irradiation. Photomed Laser Surg 22:343–350
33. de Mello ED, Pagnoncelli RM, Munin E et al (2008) Comparative histological analysis of bone healing of standardized bone defects performed with the Er:YAG laser and steel burs. Lasers Med Sci 23:253–260
34. Romeo U, Del Vecchio A, Palaia G, Tenore G, Visca P, Maggiore C (2009) Bone damage induced by different cutting instruments. An in vitro study. Braz Dent J 20:162–168
35. Vescovi P, Merigo E, Manfredi M et al (2009) Surgical treatment of maxillary osteonecrosis due to bisphosphonates using an Er:YAG (2940 nm) laser. Discussion of 17 clinical cases. Rev Belge Med Dent 64:87–95
36. Vescovi P, Manfredi M, Merigo E et al (2010) Surgical approach with Er:YAG laser on Osteonecrosis of the Jaws (ONJ) in patients under Bisphosphonate Therapy (BPT). Lasers Med Sci 25:101–113
37. Merigo E, Vescovi P, Manfredi M et al (2010) Surgical Er:YAG laser assisted treatment of BRONJ (Bisphosphonate-Related Osteonecrosis of the Jaws). Lasers Med Sci 25:S43
38. Angiero F, Sannino C, Borloni R, Crippa R, Benedicenti S, Romanos GE (2009) Osteonecrosis of the jaws caused by bisphosphonates: evaluation of a new therapeutic approach using the Er:YAG laser. Laser Med Sci 24:849–856
39. Stubinger S, Dissmann JP, Pinho NC, Saldamli B, Seitz O, Sader R (2009) A preliminary report about treatment of bisphosphonate related osteonecrosis of the jaw with Er:YAG laser ablation. Lasers Surg Med 41:28–30
40. Vescovi P, Campisi G, Fusco V et al (2011) Bisphosphonate-Related Osteonecrosis of the Jaws (BRONJ) not associated to invasive dental procedures: a retrospective analysis of 567 cases in an Italian multicenter study. Oral Oncol 47:191–194
41. Mavrokokki T, Cheng A, Stein B, Gos A (2007) Nature and frequency of bisphosphonate-associated osteonecrosis in Australia. J Oral Maxillofac Surg 65:415–423
42. Malden N, Beltes C, Lopes V (2009) Dental extractions and bisphosphonates: the assessment, consent and management, a proposed algorithm. Br Dent J 206:93–98
43. Vescovi P, Fornaini C, Merigo E et al (2009) Use of Nd:YAG laser biostimulation for dental extractions scheme in patients under bisphosphonates therapy. Lasers Med Sci 24:S44
44. Vescovi P, Nammour S (2010) Bisphosphonate-related osteonecrosis of the jaw (BRONJ) therapy. A critical review. Minerva Stomatol 59:181–213

Minimally Invasive Surgical Treatment 13

Claudio Marchetti, Gian Andrea Pelliccioni, Filippo Moretti, Francesco Saverio De Ponte, Giuseppe Lombardo and Carla Nava

Abstract

Minimally invasive surgery refers to all surgical procedures in which there is only a small incision or no incision at all. It is possible to distinguish between preventive surgery, aimed at removing actual causes that could worsen the patient's quality of life, and palliative surgery, aimed, for example, as discussed herein, at removing part of the osteonecrosis. Marsupialization of cystic lesions is appropriate if a cyst has already eroded the cortical bone. The procedure involves an incision to expose the fenestration, followed by the insertion of a small Teflon tube for draining the lesion and reducing the endocystic pressure. This creates favorable conditions for neo-apposition of the bone inside the lacunae. Apicoectomy can be performed when endodontic therapy is not sufficient to treat a granuloma; as in marsupialization, this technique is possible only if the radiographic examinations confirm the presence of a fenestration of the cortical bone. Debridement is specifically carried out to treat stage 2 lesions, in patients who experience pain due to an inflammation of the surrounding soft tissues, or when there are sharp bone spicules. Sequestrectomy is viable only if the surgeon verifies the sequestrum's mobility; it can be performed by removing the fragment atraumatically, using surgical forceps. Drug holiday is useful in patients receiving oral bisphosphonates and requiring oral surgery. Suspension of these drugs increases bone activity, which can be monitored by significant increases in CTX levels over time. A lower limit of >150 pg/ml is recommended to proceed with surgery. Piezosurgery is another minimally invasive treatment for removing necrotic tissues, creating regular bony borders. A prerequisite for these procedures is a good control of oral hygiene and antibiotic prophylaxis.

F. Moretti (✉)
Department of Oral Sciences, Unit of Oral and Maxillofacial Surgery,
S. Orsola Hospital, University of Bologna, Bologna, Italy
e-mail: filippo.moretti5@unibo.it

F. S. De Ponte (ed.), *Bisphosphonates and Osteonecrosis of the Jaw: A Multidisciplinary Approach*, DOI: 10.1007/978-88-470-2083-2_13,

13.1 Introduction

The current literature relating to the therapeutic treatment of bisphosphonate-induced osteonecrosis of the jaw (BIONJ) is far from homogeneous, although there is wide agreement about preventive strategies. A careful analysis of the literature reveals two main schools of thought: the first, which could be defined as "interventionist," is based on a surgical [1–3]; the second, which could be defined as "conservative," calls for a less invasive approach [4–11].

A position paper published by the American Association of Oral and Maxillofacial Surgeons (AAOMS) in 2009 set forth common strategies and provided surgeons with guidelines [12]. First of all, it stated the aim of treatment: preservation of the patient's quality of life by keeping secondary infections and pain under control by preventing extension of the lesion and the development of further areas of necrosis. Moreover, the AAOMS provided the following classification, using four staging categories with related therapeutic approaches:

- Stage 0: The patient does not show evident clinical signs of osteonecrosis, rather he/she might have symptoms or atypical clinical and radiographic signs. These patients do not have a recent or positive remote anamnesis of BIONJ.
- Stage 1: Exposed necrotic bone in asymptomatic patients with no clear signs of infection.
- Stage 2: Exposed necrotic bone with pain and clinical evidence of infection.
- Stage 3: Exposed necrotic bone with pain, infection, and one or more of the following: pathologic fracture, extra-oral fistula, oro-sinusal or oro-nasal communication, osteolysis extending to the inferior border or to the maxillary sinus floor, osteonecrosis extended beyond the alveolar bone tissue.

As far as the therapeutic approach is concerned, the AAOMS concluded that surgery should be postponed as much as possible and reserved for stage 3 patients only, or for those who do not respond to antibiotics therapy. More precisely, minor surgery is appropriate for patients who have a bone sequestrum with well-defined edges. A conservative approach is generally indicated for patients with stage 0, 1, or 2 BIONJ.

Vescovi et al., among others, argued that since the entire skeleton is subject to the action of bisphosphonates, identifying lesion-free edges is far from being a definitive approach to treatment, in contrast to the treatment of patients with lesions such as osteoradionecrosis [13]. In other words, even free bleeding edges, due to surgical trauma, can be subject to a relapse of the primary lesion and therefore to a new peripheral osteonecrosis. This means that, rather than being a definitive treatment, surgical therapy, while aimed at removing infected tissue, can instead cause a wider bone exposure and even an exacerbation of symptoms. Such considerations constitute the basis of all minimally invasive strategies reported in the existing literature.

13.2 Minimally Invasive Surgery

Minimally invasive surgery refers to all surgical procedures done with only a small incision or no incision at all. Two different types of minimally invasive surgery can be identified in relation to patients receiving bisphosphonate therapy:

1. Preventive surgery: aimed at removing concurrent causes which, if not adequately treated, can worsen the patient's quality of life. More precisely, there are two types of surgical procedures:
   - Extraction of non-recoverable teeth that cannot be treated conservatively or which can damage contiguous teeth or surrounding bone tissue
   - Marsupialization of cystic lesions
2. Palliative surgery: aimed at removing part of the osteonecrotic bone tissue (sequestrectomy) or the alleviation of symptoms (surgical drainage of the abscess)

A prerequisite for any surgical procedure is correct patient preparation, which will avoid the risk of infectious-inflammatory complications or a worsening of the patient's conditions. This is why it is vital to keep local and systemic bacterial contamination under control. Patients should be educated to carry out oral hygiene at home using mouth rinses together with interdental brushes and tips (if necessary). Also, they should receive frequent professional plaque removal (every 2–3 months). As previously noted, surgery should be supported by adequate antibiotic prophylaxis to minimize systemic bacterial contamination.

It goes without saying that, rather than being just a preliminary phase to surgery, a preventive approach based on oral hygiene and medical therapy is a therapeutic strategy as well. The protocol has been recommended by the AAOMS for patients with osteonecrosis of the jaws and is independent of the BIONJ classification stage.

13.2.1 Marsupialization of Cystic Lesions

Cystic lesions are pathological cavities lined by epithelium. These diverse lesions of the jaws can expand, ultimately eroding the cortical bone and involving adjacent soft tissue. Per definition, odontogenic cysts originate in tissues associated with teeth. Inflammatory cysts, with the most frequent type being malformative cysts, such as radicular cyst and keratocystic odontogenic tumor, can reach a significant size. A radicular cyst represents the evolution of an apical granuloma, i.e., an inflammatory process originating at the apex of a necrotic tooth that has not been adequately treated with endodontic therapy. The keratocystic odontogenic tumor is benign but has a potentially aggressive and infiltrating behavior, with a tendency to relapse.

Enucleation is the preferred treatment of cystic lesions. However, since trauma to bone tissues of patients receiving bisphoshonates should be avoided, marsupialazation is more appropriate if the lesion has already eroded the cortical bone. Surgery involves an incision in the cortical bone fenestration and the insertion of a

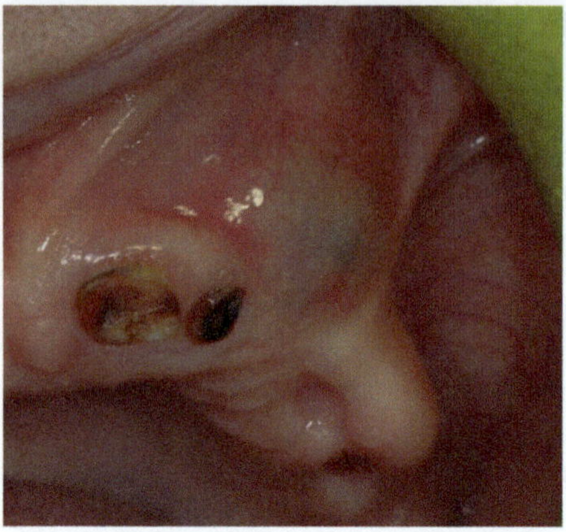

Fig. 13.1 Residual radicular cyst with an affected tooth

small Teflon tube, through which it is possible to achieve drainage of the lesion. This tube is kept in position with a non-absorbable suture. It can be used by the patient for mouth rinses with antiseptic solutions injected through an atraumatic needle. The tube allows the merging of the cystic epithelium with the mouth mucosa in approximately a week's time. This reduces the endocystic pressure and therefore creates favorable conditions for neo-apposition of the bone inside the lacunae. In the case of radicular cysts, surgery should be preceded by a correct endodontic treatment of the tooth or teeth involved (Figs. 13.1, 13.2, 13.3, 13.4).

This type of surgery should ideally be performed on soft tissues only. It is therefore crucial to analyze the bone approach surrounding the cyst with imaging techniques, such as traditional computed tomography (CT) or cone beam CT, to correctly view the presence and location of the bone erosion as a surgical access route (Figs. 13.5, 13.6, 13.7, 13.8, 13.9, 13.10).

As in the case of dental extraction, antibiotic therapy is equally recommended for marsupialization.

13.2.2 Apicoectomy

When endodontic therapy is not sufficient to treat a chronic apical granulomatous inflammatory process, an apicoectomy of the tooth can be performed, as long as the radiographic examinations confirm the presence of a fenestration of the cortical bone at the level of the root apex to be treated. It is paramount that the oral-hygiene protocol described above for tooth extraction is followed and that patients always receive antibiotic therapy (amoxicillin, metronidazole).

Apicoectomy involves lifting an over-periosteal flap, which should be sufficiently wide to allow an adequate view and should extend at least to the previous and to the following tooth. The second phase involves identifying the area of fenestration at the level of the tooth apex, after which apicoectomy can be

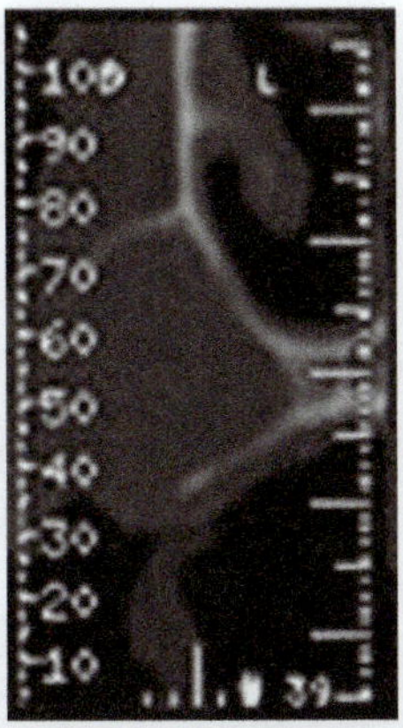

Fig. 13.2 CT Dentascan shows the presence of a cortical erosion

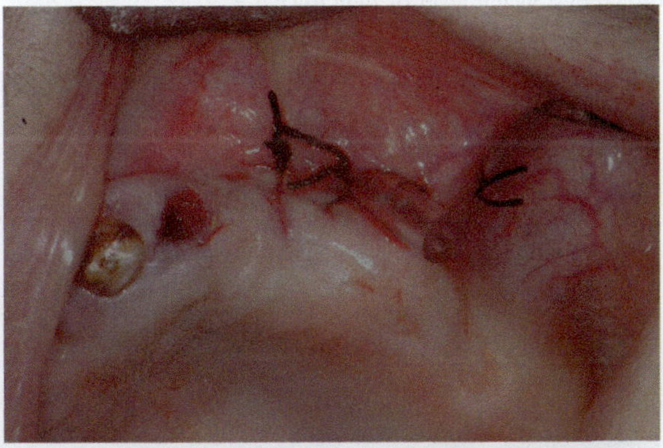

Fig. 13.3 Marsupialization of the cyst and positioning of a drainage tube

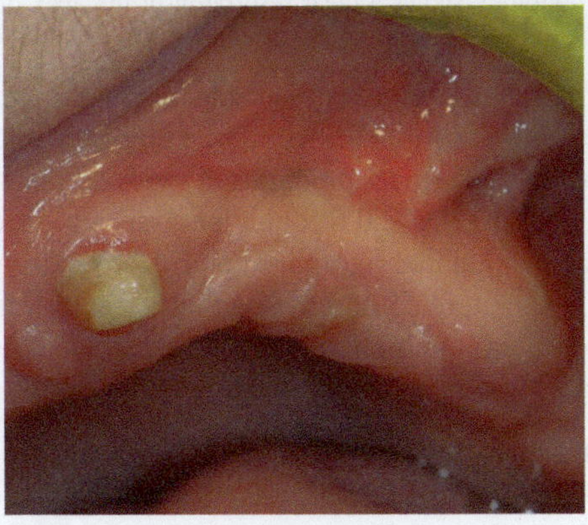

Fig. 13.4 Check-up after 6 months

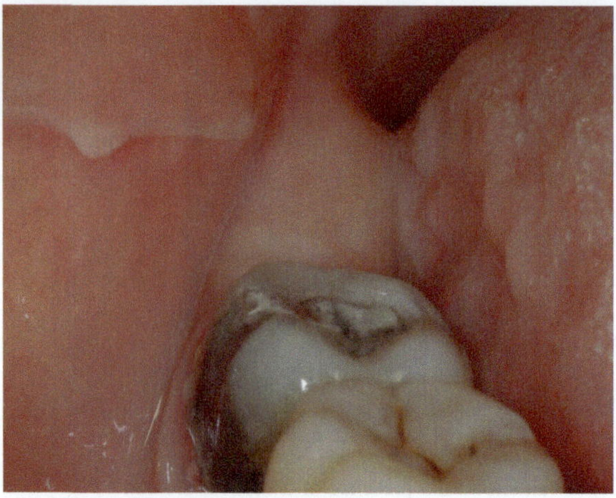

Fig. 13.5 Pericoronal cyst at the level of the crown

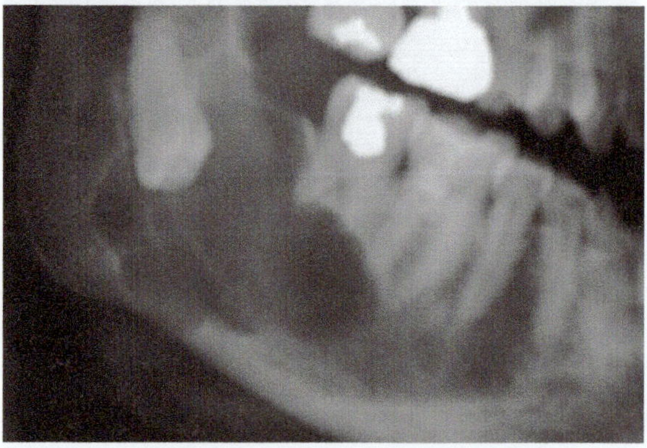

Fig. 13.6 Orthopantomography shows a clear resorption of the apex of the crowns

performed. Dental tissue is removed starting from the apex, to achieve the centralization of the radicular foramen within the diameter of the radicular section. This is followed by a retrograde preparation with ultrasonic instruments and subsequent filling. Checking the seal through methylene blue, cleaning the surgical field, and performing a final radiographic control are extremely important concluding procedures. Silk suture should be used to correctly seal the surgical injury and to prevent bacterial contamination.

13.2.3 Debridement

Debridement is a minimally invasive surgical procedure specifically carried out to treat stage 2 lesions. It is used in patients who experience pain in the osteonecrosis

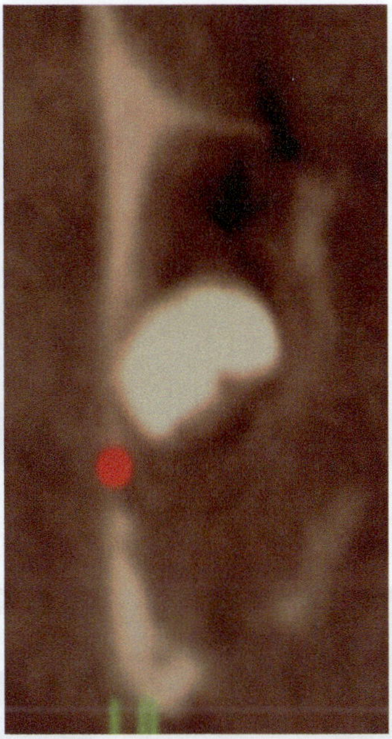

Fig. 13.7 CT Dentascan reveals erosion of the high cortical bone

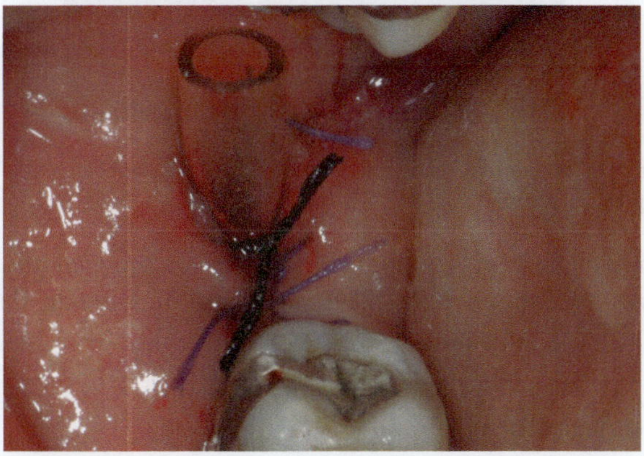

Fig. 13.8 Marsupialization of the cyst and positioning of a drainage tube

area due to an inflammation of the surrounding soft tissues, which appear erythematous and edematous after intraoral examination. This symptom is often the result of an accumulation of dental plaque and tartar above the lesion. Debridement can also be performed when there are thin sharp bone spicules, which can cause lesions by irritating the edge of the tongue. Debridement can be carried out with manual tools, such as curettes, or with ultrasonic scalers, which allow the

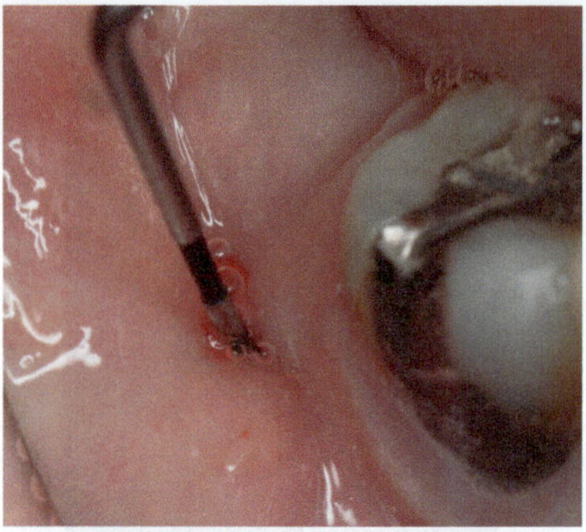

Fig. 13.9 One year after marsupialization, the lesion persists

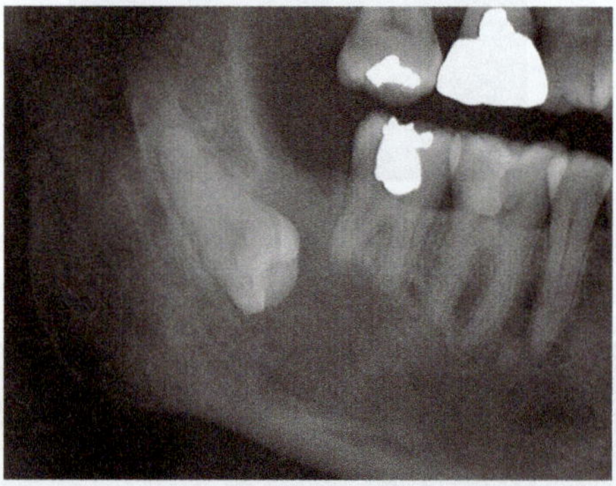

Fig. 13.10 Orthopantomography one year later shows a bone neoformation inside the cystic cavity and an apical migration

atraumatic smoothening of sharp edges. Surface cleaning of the necrotic bone tissue improves the condition of the soft tissues surrounding the necrosis and subsequently reduces the patient's symptoms.

13.2.4 Sequestrectomy

Quite often, BIONJ provokes the formation of a bone sequestrum during maintenance therapy. This is a fragment of necrotic bone tissue that first acquires mobility and then detaches from the surrounding bone. From a biological perspective, a sequestrum is the consequence of the formation of granulation tissue separating the dead bone from the underlying living bone. Detachment may affect only part of the pathological tissue, or it may lead to the removal of the entire necrotic area. In the first case, several osteonecrotic fragments detach. When the whole area detaches from the surrounding bone, there are two possible

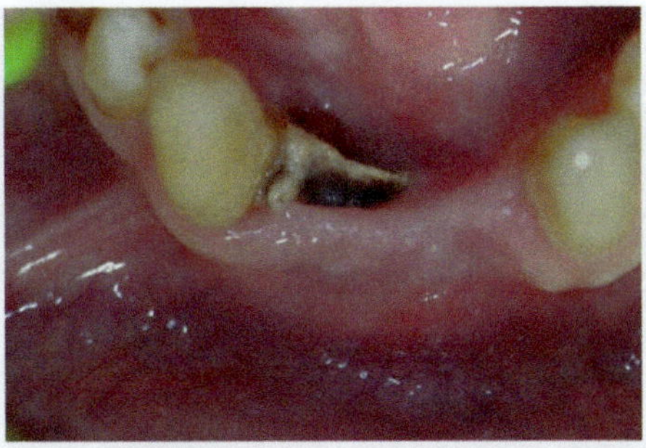

Fig. 13.11 Presence of an osteonecrotic area exposed in zones 41–42

scenarios: if the underlying tissue is healthy, a progressive and complete re-epithelialization will follow. If the underlying bone is affected by an osteitic process, a relapse will occur, rather than a complete recovery. It should be noted that the presence of healthy mucosa does not necessarily resolve the pathological process (Fig. 13.11, 13.12, 13.13, 13.14).

In some cases, after a period of exposure a bone fragment is able to move but it might not be expelled spontaneously. The surgeon's role is to verify the edges of the sequestrum, using clinical and radiographic examinations (orthopantomography, CT, MRI), and then to remove the bone fragment atraumatically using surgical forceps or Klemmer forceps.

13.2.5 Drug Holiday

Ever since the first reports on BIONJ were published in the literature, the possibility of suspending bisphosphonates has been considered, both as a preventive measure in asymptomatic patients who require maxillofacial surgery and as a therapeutic strategy, to verify whether this could somehow stimulate healing of the lesion. Neither is likely realistic in patients treated with intravenous bisphosphonates; these drugs, in fact, are typically used in oncology and play a lifesaving role. By contrast, in most cases, it should be possible to arrange with the prescribing physician a temporary suspension of oral or intramuscular bisphosphonates.

The effectiveness of a drug holiday still needs confirmations by appropriate studies; in the case reports published so far, the results have been encouraging, especially regarding the use of a drug holiday as a preventive measure. These positive findings may be related, at least in part, to the suspension of the anti-angiogenic effect, which allows better wound healing in the mucosa. However, the effects of a drug holiday upon osteoblasts and osteoclasts are still unclear, since bisphosphonates have a long half-life within the bone, such that the effectiveness of a brief suspension of therapy is questionable.

Several authors have attempted to identify objective parameters to predict the risk of osteonecrosis of the jaws. Marx proposed an index measuring the degree of bone

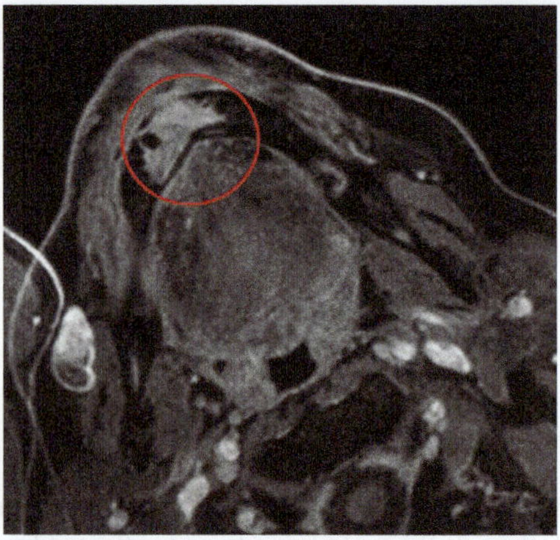

Fig. 13.12 Gadolinium MRI shows the presence of an osteonecrotic area

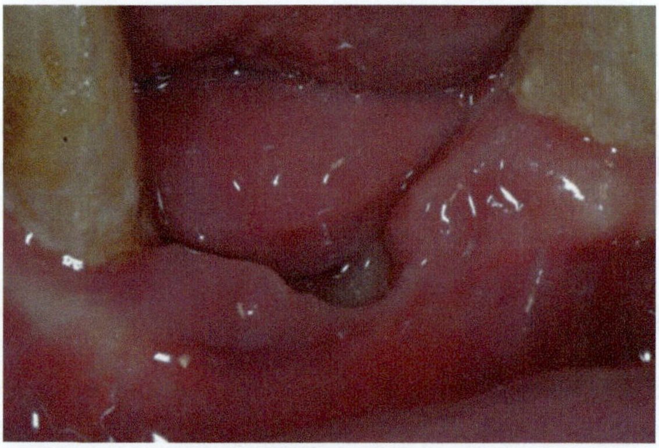

Fig. 13.13 Spontaneous detachment of an osteonecrotic sequestrum: appearance of gingival tissues. The patient had failed to properly carry out the hygienic routine recommended to every patient at the very beginning of the follow-up cycle and required further instruction to encourage compliance

remodeling that can be checked frequently and easily, by comparing serum levels before and after a drug holiday [9]. These criteria are met in the CTX test, in which a breakdown product of type I collagen is measured in serum samples. Type I collagen is the major protein in the bone tissue, representing 98% of total proteins. The β-cross-linked telopeptide CTX is released during osteoclast-mediated resorption and its level in serum is therefore proportionate to the activity of these cells. Normal CTX scores are usually above 300 pg/ml, whereas a lower score indicates various levels of suppression of bone tissue activity. Marx showed that patients with osteonecrosis have CTX levels <150 pg/ml (1 pmol/l = 0.129 pg/ml). Following bisphosphonate discontinuation for a period of 6 months, the CTX score increased significantly, by a monthly average of 25.9 pg/ml.

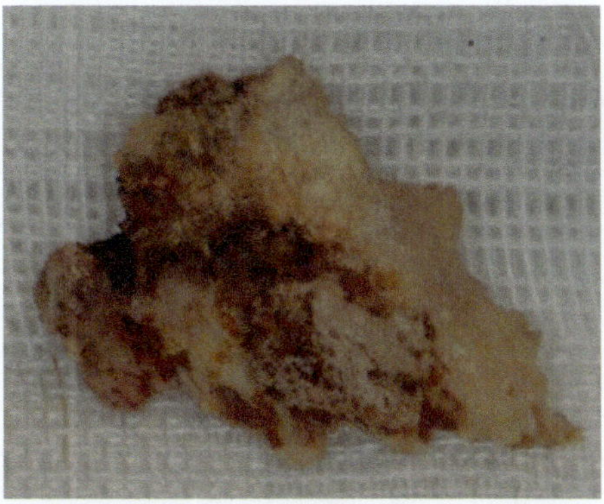

Fig. 13.14 Osteonecrotic sequestrum

These data show that an appropriate drug holiday together with monitoring of the CTX score can be a useful tool in patients receiving oral bisphosphonates but requiring oral surgery. A lower limit of >150 pg/ml is recommended to proceed with surgery while limiting the risks of complications. If this level is not achieved, then, in agreement with the treating physician, patients can take a drug holiday of 4–6 months, after which the test should be repeated (Fig. 13.15). It has been shown that, if the degree of bone mineralization reaches a plateau after oral or intramuscular intake of bisphosphonates, a drug holiday does not induce further changes, even if extended for another 6 months. It is currently recommended that patients who have been receiving bisphosphonates together with corticosteroids for at least 3 years should take a drug holiday from the bisphosphonate 3 months before surgery and continuing until the bone recovery is complete [12].

There is a wide range of opinions concerning the suspension of bisphosphonate treatment in patients with BIONJ. Most data support the discontinuation of oral or intramuscular bisphosphonates as a contributing factor in the recovery from complications, whereas it is generally agreed that the discontinuation of intravenous bisphosphonates offers no benefit (it is not an option since in these cases the drugs life-saving).

13.3 Minimally Invasive Surgery Using the Piezoelectric Drill

Surgical treatment of BIONJ should be limited to stage III patients (pain, infection, fistula, pathological fractures) and consists of a sequestrectomy of the involved region within radiologically healthy margins [14]. The procedure can be performed under local or general anesthesia depending on the extent of the affected area. Initially, treatment consisted of a minimal debridement of the exposed bone combined with antibiotics and hyperbaric therapy but this proved to be unsuitable due to the exacerbation of symptoms [15–17].

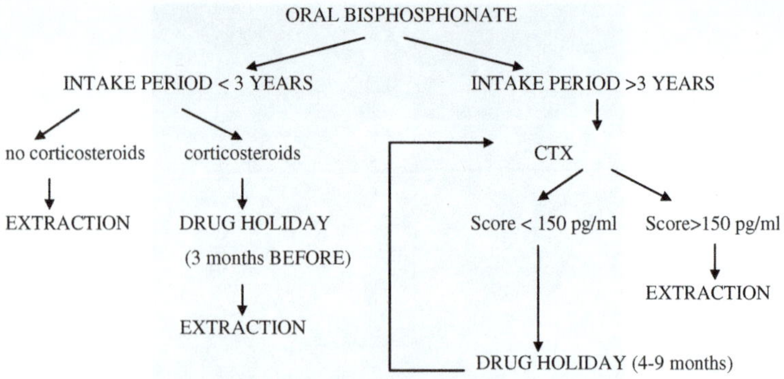

Fig. 13.15 Protocol for tooth extractions in patients treated with oral bisphosphonates

In order to ensure a full recovery, the following rules must be applied [16]:

1. Removal of all hard and soft necrotic tissue
2. Elimination of any granulation tissue; repair of the fistula
3. Restoration of tissue continuity to minimize contact between saliva and bone

A normal blood supply of the bony and soft tissues that surround the necrotic bone may be an important factor in the success rate of surgical treatment for BIONJ.

The most influential surgical factor for recovery is removal of the necrotic tissue, creating regular bony borders. It is important to smooth off any sharp bony spurs because, since BIONJ patients have a reduced potential for bone remodeling, the soft tissue must lie on smooth bone. The adjacent teeth are removed if they lie <1 cm from the borders of resection. A tension-free closure of the mucosa is essential to promote soft-tissue healing.

In addition, surgery must be accompanied by a suitable antibiotic regimen. Broad-spectrum antibiotics are administered intravenously for a week. If any purulence is observed during surgery, antibiotics are continued orally for a brief period (10–15 days) [18]. It should be noted that an incomplete curettage will lead to persistence of the BIONJ, which may be wrongly attributed to resistance to antibiotic therapy [17].

An innovative surgical procedure that further reduces damage to both the bone tissue and the soft tissue surrounding areas of osteonecrosis has been advantageously employed in the management of BIONJ patients. Piezoelectric surgery was only recently introduced into oral surgery but its traumatic impact was quickly confirmed to be less than that of traditional surgery. This technique employs ultrasonic vibrations that make it possible to cut only the bone, without damaging the soft tissues, because the cutting action is blocked when the drill comes into contact with non-mineralized tissues [19]. Consequently, there is a far lower risk of iatrogenic lesions of the adjacent tissues [20].

The piezoelectric drill allows precise and safe osteotomies [19, 21, 22]. The physical principle on which it is based is the transduction of ultrasound waves, which are obtained by contracting and expanding the piezoelectric ceramic in an

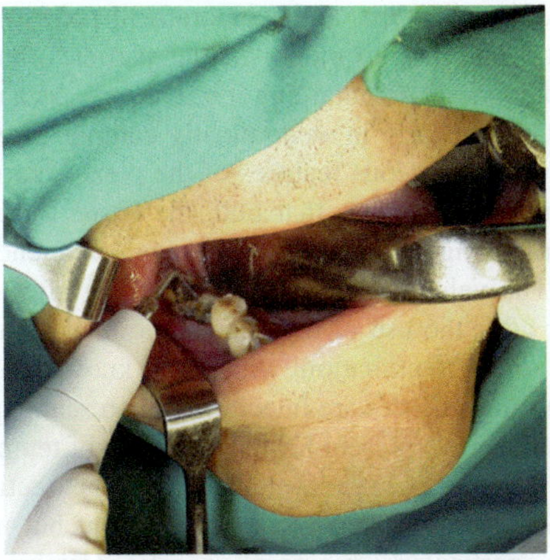

Fig. 13.16 Piezosurgery appliances

electric field (indirect piezoelectric effect) [18, 20, 21]. The vibrations are amplified and transferred onto the module of the drill. Applying the drill to bone with light pressure while irrigating the tissue with saline solution triggers cavitation, resulting in cutting of the mineralized tissues alone (Fig. 13.16) [21, 22].

Compared to traditional cutting instruments, the piezoelectric drill offers the following advantages:

- The possibility of micrometric cutting, because the drill-point vibrates with a modulated frequency of ultrasound that constantly keeps the bone clean during cutting and avoids excessively high temperatures.
- Selective and safe cutting, as the vibration frequency is optimized for mineralized tissues (to cut soft tissues, different frequencies are required) [21, 23, 24]. However, following any contact with soft tissues, cutting should be interrupted immediately to avoid unnecessary thermal stress [21].

Traditional drilling produces a cutting action that combines velocity and twisting of the drill with the pressure impressed on the handle. These features make it less safe to use than piezoelectric drilling [21]. Surgical control of the piezoelectric drill requires less force because no extra force is needed to counteract the rotation and oscillation of the device [19, 24]. Furthermore, the contamination of bone by metal that may occur after traditional drilling can lead to structural bone alterations and a toxic effect on living cells [23].

In an osteotomy starting from the cortical bone and carried out with the traditional drill, the amount of force employed can suddenly become excessive when the drill reaches the spongiosa. The resulting immediate loss of control can be extremely dangerous to delicate anatomical structures, such as vessels and nerves, located in the vicinity of the surgical site [21].

In contrast to the use of micro- and standard drill points, ultrasonic vibrations break up the irrigation liquid into much smaller particles that are then projected away from the operative field, maintaining it blood-free. As a result, intraoperative control is far better, particularly in anatomically complex areas.

Among the many advantageous features of the piezoelectric drill in surgery to treat BIONJ, the most important is that both the tissue treated and the adjacent tissue maintain their healing potential even after high-frequency sound waves have been applied [20]. The velocity of bone tissue healing after osteotomy has been shown to be higher after the use of a piezoelectric drill than after an oscillating drill because there is no inflammation, which is a known cause of delayed bone regeneration. The cutting surfaces are intact, do not present gaps or fragments, and vital osteocytes and fibrin are present [21]. The effects of temperature increases on the cutting surface have also been evaluated. In bone sections examined after piezoelectric drilling, necrotic phenomena were absent but nucleated osteocytes and growth factors, particularly biomorphogenetic proteins indicative of early bone regeneration, were visible. In BIONJ patients, use of the piezoelectric drill reduces mechanical stress on the surrounding soft tissues as well as on the bone itself, since surgical trauma is kept to a minimum. Soft tissues are known to be able to heal as long as the underlying bone is smooth and infection-free. One of the main disadvantages of the piezoelectric drill, described in the literature, is an increase in the duration of surgery [21].

Patients surgically treated with the piezoelectric drill underwent follow-up examinations 1, 2 weeks, and 1, 3, 6, and 12 months after surgery. Evaluation focused mainly on: pain (Visual Analogue Scale 0–10), clinical features (healing of intraoral soft tissues), and instrumental investigations (panoramic X-ray at 3, 6 and 12 months post-operatively; CT-scan of the maxillary-facial bones at 6 and 12 months post-operatively).

The success of the surgical procedures is defined radiographically as the absence of bone disruption in the surgical area and the integrity of the mucosa for atleast 12 months. Resolution of painful symptoms is considered a less reliable index of success after resection. Instead, the absence or significant reduction of painful symptoms indicates that the BIONJ has been properly managed, while refractory pain indicates that resection was only marginally successful.

References

1. Pancholi M, Edwards A, Langton S (2007) Bisphosphonate induced osteochemonecrosis of the jaw mimicking a tumour. Br Dent J 203(2):87–89
2. Bedogni A, Saia G, Ragazzo M, Betini G et al (2007) Bisphosphonate-associated osteonecrosis can hide jaw mestastases. Bone 41(6):942–945
3. Montazeri AH, Erskine J, McQuaker I (2007) Oral sodium clodronate induced osteonecrosis of the jaw in a patient with myeloma. Eur J Haemtol 79:69–71
4. Ferrari S, Bianchi B, Savi A, Poli T, Multinu A, Balestreri A, Ferri A (2008) Fibula free flap with endosseous implants for reconstructing a resected mandible in bisphosphonate osteonecrosis. J Oral Maxillofac Surg 66:999–1003

5. Lehrer S, Montazem A, Ramanathan L, Pessin-Minsley M, Pfail J, Stock R, Kogan R (2008) Normal serum bone markers in bisphosphonate-induced osteonecrosis of the jaws. Oral Surg Oral Med Oral Pathol Oral Radiol 106(3):389–391
6. Ficarra G, Beninati F, Rubino I, Vannucchi A, Longo G, Tonelli P, Pini Prato G (2005) Osteonecrosis of the jaws in periodontal patients with a history of bisphosphonates treatment. J Clin Period 32:1123–1128
7. Freiberger J, Padilla-Burgos R, Chhoeu A, Kraft K, Boneta O, Moon RE, Piantadosi C (2007) Hyperbaric oxygen treatment and bisphosphonate-induced osteonecrosis of the jaw: a case series. J Oral Maxillofac Surg 65:1321–1327
8. Magopoulos C, Karakinaris G, Telioudis Z, Vahtsevanos K, Dimitrakopoulos I, Antoniadis K, Delaroudis S (2007) Osteonecrosis of the jaws due to bisphosphonate use. A review of 60 cases and treatment proposals. Am J Otolaryng 28:158–163
9. Marx RE, Cillo J, Ulloa J (2007) Oral bisphosphonate-induced osteonecrosis: risk factors, prediction of risk using serum CTX testing, prevention and treatment. J Oral Maxillofac Surg 65:2397–2410
10. Lazarovici TS, Yahalom R, Taicher S, Elad S, Hardan I, Yarom N (2009) Bisphosphonate-related osteonecrosis of the jaws: a single-center study of 101 patients. J Oral Maxillofac Surg 67(4):850–855
11. Montebugnoli L, Felicetti L, Gissi D, Pizzigallo A, Pelliccioni GA, Marchetti C (2007) Bisphosphonate-associated osteonecrosis can be controlled by non-surgical management. Oral Surg Oral Med Oral Pathol Oral Radiol 104:473–477
12. Ruggiero SL, Dodson TB, Assael LA, Landesberg R, Marx RE, Mehrotra B (2009) American Association of Oral and Maxillofacial Surgeons position paper on bisphosphonate-related osteonecrosis of the jaws-2009 update. J Oral Maxillofac Surg 67:2–12
13. Vescovi P, Nammour S (2010) Bisphosphonate-related osteonecrosis of the jaw (BRONJ) therapy. A critical review. Minerva Stomat 59(4):181–213
14. Vescovi P, Merigo E, Mandredi M et al (2010) Surgical approach with Er.YAG laser on osteonecrosis of the jaws (ONJ) in patients under bisphosphonate therapy (BPT). Lasers Med Sci 25:101–113
15. Adornato MC, Morocs I, Rozanski J (2007) The treatment of bisphosphonate-associated osteonecrosis of the jaws with bone resection and autologous platelet-derived growth factors. J Am Dent Assoc 138:971–977
16. Tirelli G, Biasotto M, Chiandussi S et al (2009) Bisphosphonate-associated osteonecrosis of the jaws: the limits of a conservative approach. Head Neck 31:1249–1254
17. Alons K, Kuijpers SCC, de Jong EE, van Merkesteyn JPR (2007) Treating low- and medium-potency bisphosphonate-related osteonecrosis of the jaws with a protocol for the treatment of chronic suppurative osteomyelitis: report of 7 cases. Oral Surg Oral Med Oral Pathol Oral Radiol Endod 107:1–7
18. Kademani D, Koka S, Lacy MQ, Rajkumar V (2006) Primary surgical therapy for osteonecrosis of the jaw secondary to bisphosphonate therapy. Mayo Clin Proc 81(8):1100–1103
19. Bains VK, Mohan R, Bairns R (2008) Application of ultrasound in periodontics: Part II. J Indian Soc Periodontol 12(3):55–61
20. Barone A, Santini S, Maconini S et al (2008) Osteotomy and membrane elevation during the maxillary sinus augmentation procedure A comparative study: piezoelectric device vs. conventional rotative instruments. Clin Oral Impl Res. 19:511–515
21. Crosetti E, Battison B, Succo G (2009) Piezosurgery in head and neck oncological and reconstructive surgery: personal experience on 127 cases. Acta Otorhinolaryngol Ital 29:1–9
22. Muñoz-Guerra MF, Naval Gas L, Capote Moreno A (2009) Le Fort I osteotomy, bilateral sinus lift, and inlay bone-grafting for reconstruction in the severely atrophic maxilla: a new vision of the sandwich technique, using bone scrapers and piezosurgery. J Oral Maxillofac Surg 67:613–618

23. Chiriac G, Herten M, Schwarz F, Rothamel D, Becker J (2005) Autogenous bone chips: influence of a new piezoelectric device (Piezosurgerys) on chip morphology, cell viability and differentiation. J Clin Periodontol 32:994–999
24. Degerliyurt K, Akar V, Denizci S, Yucel E (2009) Bone lid technique with piezosurgery to preserve inferior alveolar nerve. Oral Surg Oral Med Oral Pathol Oral Radiol Endod 108:1–5

14 Major Surgery in BIONJ

Luciano Catalfamo, Carla Nava, Giuseppe Lombardo
and Francesco Saverio De Ponte

Abstract

Major surgery in BIONJ should be considered only for patients with stage III disease and large lesions. In this chapter, the characteristics of patients who are candidates for major surgery are described. We also discuss the methods used in jawbone resection, reconstruction of secondary defects, and the resolution of complications in advanced-stage disease.

14.1 Introduction

Ever since osteonecrosis of the jaw was associated with the use of bisphosphonates therapy, there has been an attempt to establish standard treatment protocols. However, this has not been entirely possible since patients with bisphosphonates-induced osteonecrosis of the jaw (BIONJ) have a less predictable reaction to surgery than is the case with patients having other types of osteonecrosis, such as radiation-induced osteonecrosis, osteomyelitis, or osteitis caused by infection or trauma [1–7]. Indeed, the previous literature revealed a common concern that surgery could cause further osteonecrosis. Instead, treatment aims to eliminate pain, control the infection of the bone and soft tissues, and minimize the progression of necrosis [2, 8], Nonetheless, the primary aim is prevention, using chlorhexidine oral rinses, systemic antibiotics, and protection of the site from further trauma. Conservative treatment and sequestrectomy are performed in the

F. S. De Ponte (✉)
Unit of Maxillo-Facial Surgery,
University of Messina, Messina, Italy
e-mail: deponte.francescosaverio7@gmail.com

F. S. De Ponte (ed.), *Bisphosphonates and Osteonecrosis of the Jaw: A Multidisciplinary Approach*, DOI: 10.1007/978-88-470-2083-2_14,

early stages as needed and using atraumatic tools, such as the piezoelectric drill [9–16]. Surgery is usually reserved for the most serious cases, such as stage III disease, and in symptomatic patients with large lesions [10, 17].

While previously it was believed that obtaining vital bone tissue margins was difficult, since the entire jaw is affected by bisphosphonates, it was recently demonstrated that this is not the case [18, 19]. In 2006, Ruggiero argued that vascularized or non-vascularized bone flap reconstruction should be avoided in BIONJ patients, given the risk of induced necrosis [2, 19]. Nocini et al. and Bedogni et al. [19, 20] examined surgical specimens of resected jaws together with margins of bone resection. Histological analysis of the tissue confirmed the diagnosis of BIONJ while an analysis of bone resection margins identified areas of normal bone architecture. These data suggested that BIONJ recurrence is caused by the presence of normal bone in resection margins rather than by the reconstruction method itself [19, 20].

Candidates for surgery are patients with no clinical conditions preventing surgery and: stage III lesions, marked by exposed bone and painful adjacent soft tissues; acute infection that cannot be treated with oral or endovenous antibiotics; extraoral fistula; or pathological fracture or wide osteolysis leading to fracture [2, 8, 21].

Surgery might require a temporary suspension of chemotherapy; however, this is not possible in some patients [18]. Otherwise, patients should not receive bisphosphonates for at least 2 months before surgery, in agreement with oncologists [7, 18, 21–23] and as recommended by Marx (2003) and Ruggiero (2006) [2]. Although suspension of bisphosphonates was later considered irrelevant due to their long half-life, this protocol has been retained given the success rate of the overall surgical approach. The American Association of Oral and Maxillofacial Surgeons (AAOMS) suggests a 3-month pre-operative suspension for patients who have received oral bisphosphonates for more than 3 years or who have simultaneously taken corticosteroids [18].

According to Carlson, patients who have received oral bisphosphonates are those who benefit most from mandibular resection, with successful maxillectomy demonstrated in patients receiving oral and endovenous bisphosphonates [24].

14.2 Surgical Protocol

As noted above, in BIONJ patients may not benefit from aggressive surgery of bone defects since it can cause the progression of necrosis. Therefore, a more conservative approach is commonly recommended [8, 25, 26]. However, when patients do not respond to conservative treatment and there is disease progression, the only possible solution is major surgery [8, 21], with computed tomography (CT) or magnetic resonance imaging (MRI) used pre-operatively to identify the precise extension of the disease [18].

Ruggiero et al. were the first to suggest a lesion staging system, with recommendations for treatment according to disease stage [2]. Accordingly, surgery was successful in 85% of patients with advanced stage disease, with better results

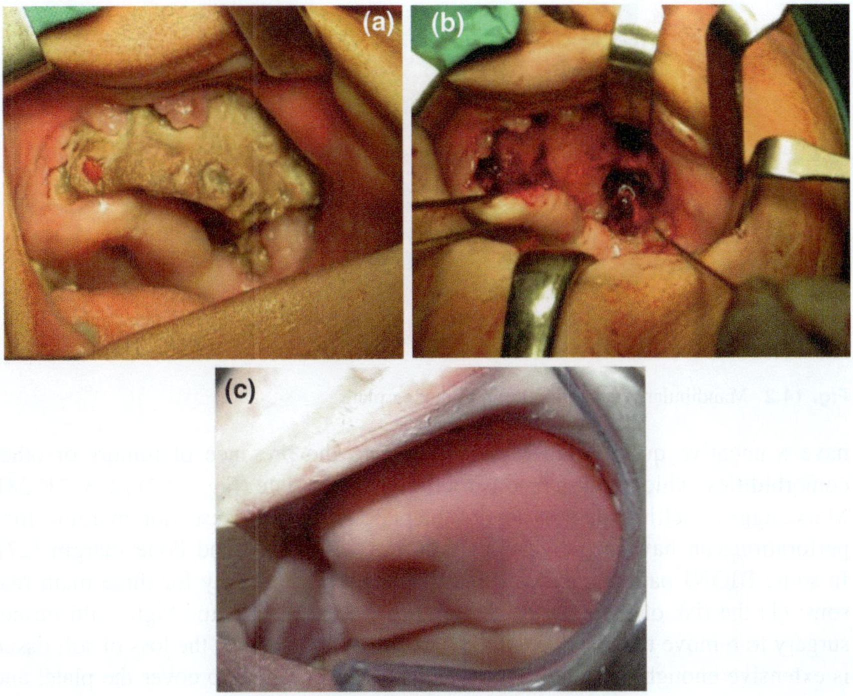

Fig. 14.1 **a** Preoperative view of lesion. **b** Postoperative oro-antral communication. **c** Maxillary obturator

achieved using a superior mandibular resection than a marginal or segmental resection [2, 17].

Resection of refractory BIONJ takes into account: (1) that the disease originates and is more serious in the alveolar bone and (2) that it is limited to the jaw [27]. Bone resection margins should be 1 cm beyond the margins of the osteomyelitic process, as identified on pre-operative CT or MRI [17, 28]. This is why resection should not extend beyond the infraorbital foramen nor involve the pterygoids, nasal septum, or orbital frame. Since bone exposure also necessitates significant soft-tissue loss, most mandibular resections lead to an oro-antral nasal communication, which in turn requires the use of a maxillary obturator (Fig. 14.1). An oro-antral nasal communications can be closed with a Bichat flap when the defect is small or with a temporalis muscle flap in the case of a large defect [27].

Carlson performed marginal mandibular resections in patients whose clinical and X-ray examinations revealed necrotic bone isolated from the alveolar portion. Segmental resection was carried out when the lesion was more extended or in patients with an orocutaneous fistula [24].

When BIONJ causes a pathological fracture, the affected part of the jaw is resected, a reconstruction plate is inserted, and no bone reconstruction is performed, since the remaining part of the jaw is extremely thin and most patients

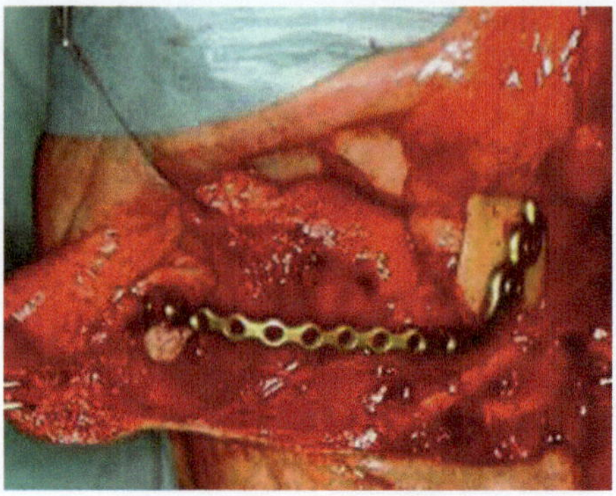

Fig. 14.2 Mandibular reconstruction with locking plate

have a negative quod vitam prognosis due to the presence of tumors or other comorbidities, which makes reconstruction inappropriate (Fig. 14.2) [2, 3, 21, 28]. Marx suggests setting the first hole of the plate close to the resection margin, since perforation can have negative effects on the periosteum and bone margin [27]. In some BIONJ patients, plates cannot be inserted, generally for three main reasons: (1) the risk of secondary infection around the plate is too high, with further surgery to remove the plate causing the loss of soft tissue; (2) the loss of soft tissue is extensive enough that there is insufficient healthy tissue to cover the plate, and the patient is not a candidate for flap surgery; (3) the patient is very weak due to chemotherapy. In these cases, surgery should be brief and limited, with the insertion of a plate, if any, postponed to a period when the patient's systemic condition and that of the local tissue improve. Nasogastric tubes or tracheostomy are not usually necessary in these cases as most patients adapt to the resulting malocclusion; however, they become necessary in the case of resection of the mandibular symphisis along the midline [27].

Bone reconstruction of the surgical defects is uncommon because the anesthesiological risks for oncology patients are high and the fact that after resection and the insertion of a reconstruction plate the pain disappears and a good functional recovery follows. In addition, in patients with multiple myeloma, bone reconstruction is not recommended because of the risk of medullary involvement [27].

Very little has been published on the role of the free fibula flap in the treatment of BIONJ [17]. Also, vascularized bone reconstruction is not recommended for BIONJ patients due to the risk of necrosis in the treated area [19]. Coletti, in 2008 [28], described a case of pseudoarthrosis that occurred after a bone graft and argued that the traditional surgical approach of flap reconstruction was not appropriate due to the risk of a necrotic bone at the resection margins [8, 21]. Local pedunculated flaps have been used for patients with a large mucosal dehiscence or bone sequestrum. In those sites that are amenable to local tissue transfer, a Bichat flap can be rotated in the surgical defect to facilitate closure without tension in the margins; the donor site mucosalizes secondarily [3]. Tirelli et al. [8] described a case of mandibular bone resection on healthy margins, followed by reconstruction with a plate and using a lobed skin flap and the platysma muscle to cover the surgical wound. As explained by those authors, flap collocation was not successful since it resulted in fistula formation and dehiscence within the flap [8].

According to Engroff, in many cases the area of bone involvement is well defined and it is possible to obtain margins of vital bone. While it is true that surgery can lead to further bone necrosis, this does not mean that the disease cannot be treated [17].

In many patients with stage III disease, there is a significant loss of mucosa and/or skin due to the anti-angiogenic effect of bisphosphonates, and above all because of long-term secondary infections, which lyse the soft tissues and provoke subcutaneous soft-tissue fibrosis. Therefore, it is important to assess the degree of soft-tissue loss, the extension of fibrosis, and the potential presence of fistulas to determine whether a flap is necessary. Generally speaking, the loss of soft-tissue and fibrosis is higher than expected [27].

14.2.1 Pectoralis Major Myocutaneous Flap

If after the insertion of a reconstruction plate an insufficient closure, or a closure under tension or without tension but with fibrotic tissue is performed, the exposed plate can lead to an open wound, with subsequent infection and the need for further surgery. The most commonly used flap is the pectoralis major myocutaneous flap based on its speed of application, allowance of adequate blood flow, and the transfer of sufficient tissue to replace large quantities of soft tissue (Fig. 14.3). The three main pedicles (thoracoacromial, thoracic, and high thoracic) are retained. In male patients, an oblique incision is often performed in order to gain access to the muscle, while a lateral approach in the inframammary fold is used in female patients in order to cover the incision and preserve the breast contour. With both incisions, a skin paddle is placed medially below the nipple at the origin of the pectoralis major, towards the lateral margin of the sternum at the junction of the sixth rib. The skin paddle and the muscle fascia are sutured at the same time to prevent lesions to capillaries. The muscle is then detached from ribs 6, 5, and 4 (in this order), and from the lateral margin of the sternum to include the medial third of the clavicle. The tendon insertion is sectioned and the flap is placed through the neck on a subplatysma level [27].

14.2.2 Trapezius Myocutaneous Flap

When the pectoral flap is not the best solution, due, for example, to a mammary prosthesis, previous chest surgery or thoracic trauma, or large breasts, the closest flap is the trapezius myocutaneous flap, which is based on the transverse cervical artery and vein. The 6-cm rule is important since the skin paddle needs to be

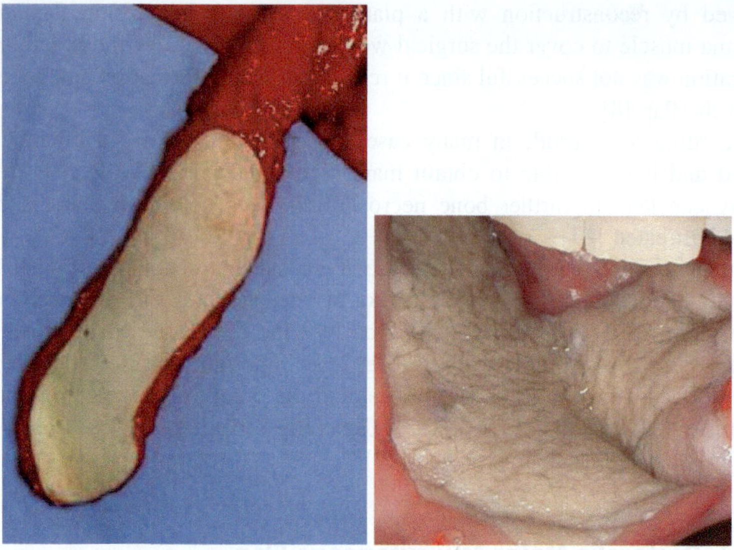

Fig. 14.3 A pectoralis major myocutaneous flap

adjacent to the midline of the back and its diameter should not be more than 6 cm below the lower point of the scapula, with the forearm in a neutral position. The flap extends backwards from the neck half way between the midline and the mid margin of the scapula. This flap requires a half-turn rotation in order to be placed in the defect so as not to affect blood flow [27].

14.2.3 Sternocleidomastoid Muscle Flap

When a primary closure is not possible and the soft-tissue in the rear jaw is limited, a pedicled sternocleidomastoid muscle flap can be placed. This flap is based entirely on the occipital vascular system while the inferior thyroid system must be sectioned to rotate the flap around the mastoid; the superior thyroid system is usually sacrificed. Nevertheless, this flap maintains sufficient blood flow to replace the soft tissues of the mandibular ramus at the labial commissure. A submandibular incision is used to gain access to the osteonecrotic lesion, together with a parallel supraclavicular incision. The sternocleidomastoid muscle is first detached from the sternal and clavicular insertions, then separated from the anterior and posterior fascia and lifted from the carotid sheath in the deepest tissues. This dissection progresses above the exit point of the spinal accessory nerve. While this exit point limits the rotation arc, in most cases it is sufficient to reach defects located behind the labial commissure. If a further rotation arc is necessary, the nerve must be rotated. Each vital muscle exposed to the oral cavity will undergo re-epithelization [24].

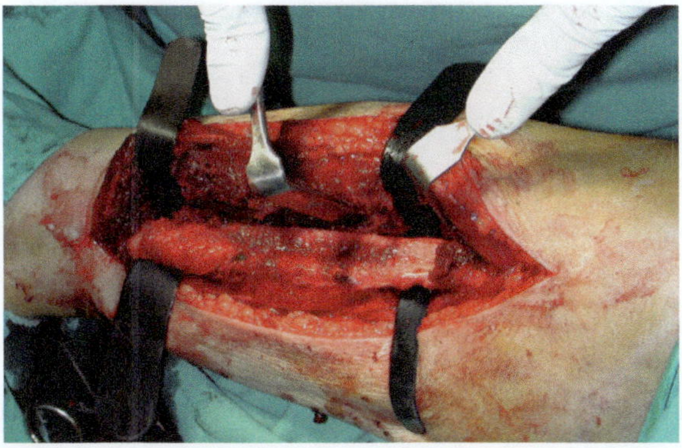

Fig. 14.4 Harvesting of a free fibula flap

14.2.4 Radial Fasciocutaneous Flap

The reconstruction of a defect of the hard palate is carried out using a free radial forearm fasciocutaneous flap, with an adequate vascular pedicle to reach facial veins in the submandibular triangle of the neck. The vascular pedicle is passed through a tunnel in the soft palate, then through the sheath, and up to the facial artery and vein, where a microvascular anastomosis is performed [17].

14.2.5 Microsurgical Reconstruction

The controversy surrounding microsurgical reconstruction is related to the fact that the occurrence of BIONJ is at least ten times higher in neoplasia patients than in osteoporosis patients. This means that most patients requiring microsurgical reconstruction are in poor health and have a limited life expectancy. The duration of microsurgical reconstruction procedures, as well as the comorbidity implied by the cancer, can compromise the immune response and delay recovery. Consequently, patients are at high risk of perioperative complications and at risk of losing the flap [19].

The iliac crest, fibula, and scapula are favorite donor sites of vascularized bone for mandibular reconstruction [19, 29]. However, the fibula is rarely the site of a metastatic bone disease or multiple myeloma, whereas the ileum and the scapula, which are rich in bone marrow, are usually involved. Accordingly, in addition to its length, which makes it an ideal flap, the fibula is the first option for subtotal mandibular reconstruction in BIONJ patients. The free fibula flap is mostly taken using a lateral approach in the anterior compartment of the leg (Fig. 14.4). The muscle cuff from the tibialis posterior and soleus is harvested with the fibula flap to repair the mucosal defect while a skin paddle is used for the reconstruction of any cutaneous defects remaining after fistula resection. Nocini et al. [19] recommended

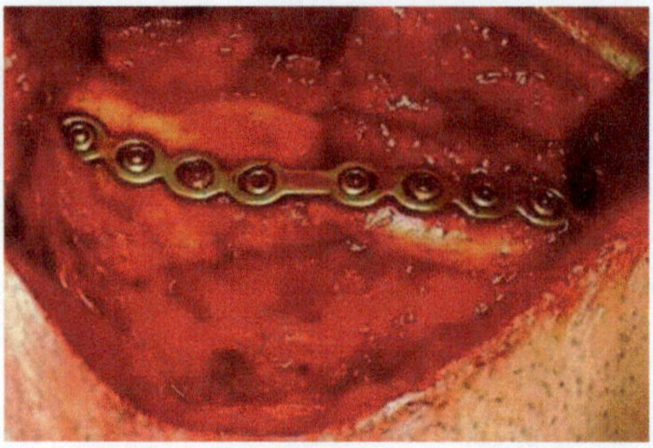

Fig. 14.5 Intra-operative view of a mandibular reconstruction with a free fibula flap

pre-operative sessions of hyperbaric oxygen therapy (HBO). Moreover, a stereolithographic model can be useful to simplify the countour of the fibula. It also allows careful planning of the resection and reconstruction, contributes to reducing the length of surgery, leads to successful functional and aesthetic results, and limits the need for secondary corrective procedures. Microvascular anastomosis is performed between the facial artery and the peroneal artery and between the venae comitantes and the tributaries of the external and internal jugular vein (Fig. 14.5) [19].

Post-operatively, endovenous antibiotic therapy for 10 days is recommended. Since the infected bone is totally removed during surgery, long-term antibiotic therapy is not required [19, 30]. Complete recovery is acknowledged when there is no exposed bone, mucosal erythema, swelling, or secretion and the surgical site is asymptomatic [18].

14.3 Follow-Up

Clinical and radiological assessments are performed 3, 6, and 12 months after surgery and every 6 months thereafter. The reconstructed bone is assessed for the development of oral mucosa sinus tracks, exposure, and purulent discharge. Orofacial pain can be assessed by comparing the pre- and post-operative visual analog scale (VAS) scores (range: 1–10). Panoramic radiographs and CT scans allow bone healing to be monitored and the detection of early signs of increased medullary bone density suggestive of BIONJ recurrence [19].

In a series reported by Nocini et al. [19], patients with fibula reconstruction recovered completely 2 months after surgery. Halitosis and pain disappeared, oral sensation was restored 14 days after surgery, and the recipient site healed without complications (pre-operative VAS 8–10, post-operative 0–2) [19].

References

1. Vieillard MH, Maes JM, Penel G et al (2008) Thirteen cases of jaw osteonecrosis in patients on bisphosphonate therapy. Jt Bone Spine 75:34–40
2. Ruggiero SL, Fantasia J, Carlson E (2006) Bisphosphonate-related osteonecrosis of the jaw: background and guidelines for diagnosis, staging and management. Oral Surg Oral Med Oral Pathol Oral Radiol Endod 102:433–441
3. Kademani D, Koka S, Lacy MQ, Rajkuma SV (2006) Primary surgical therapy for osteonecrosis of the jaw secondary to bisphosphonate therapy. Mayo Clin Proc 81(8):1100–1103
4. Bedogni A, Saia G, Ragazzo M et al (2007) Bisphosphonate-associated osteonecrosis can hide jaw metastases. Bone 41:942–945
5. Ferrari S, Bianchi B, Savi A et al (2008) Fibula free flap with endosseous implants for reconstructing a resected mandible in bisphosphonate osteonecrosis. J Oral Maxillofac Surg 66:999–1003
6. Longobardi G, Boniello R, Gasparini G, Pagano I, Pelo S (2007) Surgical therapy for osteonecotic lesions of the jaws in patients in therapy with bisphosphonates. J Craniofac Surg 18(5):1012–1017
7. Krueger CD, West PM, Sargent M, Lodolce AE, Pickard AS (2007) Bisphosphonate-induced osteonecrosis of the jaw. Ann Pharmacother 41(2):276–284
8. Tirelli G, Biasotto M, Chiandussi S et al (2009) Bisphosphonate-associated osteonecrosis of the jaws: the limits of a conservative approach. Head Neck. doi:10.1002/hed
9. Vassiliou V, Tselis N, Kardamakis D (2010) Osteonecrosis of the jaws: clinicopathologic and radiologic characteristics, preventive and therapeutic strategies. Strahlenther Onkol 186(7):367–373
10. Williamson RA (2010) Surgical management of bisphosphonate induced osteonecrosis of the jaws. Int J Oral Maxillofac Surg 39(3):251–255
11. Rustemeyer J, Bremerich A (2010) Bisphosphonate-associated osteonecrosis of the jaw: what do we currently know? A survey of knowledge given in the recent literature. Clin Oral Investig 14(1):59–64
12. Stockmann P, Vairaktaris E, Wehrhan F et al (2010) Osteotomy and primary wound closure in bisphosphonate-associated osteonecrosis of the jaw: a prospective clinical study with 12 months follow-up. Support Care Cancer 18(4):449–460
13. Khan AA, Sándor GK, Dore E et al (2009) Bisphosphonate associated osteonecrosis of the jaw. J Rheumatol 36(3):478–490
14. Alons K, Kuijpers SC, de Jong E, van Merkesteyn JP (2009) Treating low- and medium-potency bisphosphonate-related osteonecrosis of the jaws with a protocol for the treatment of chronic suppurative osteomyelitis: report of 7 cases. Oral Surg Oral Med Oral Pathol Oral Radiol Endod 107(2):e1–e7
15. 'Diego R, D'Orto O, Pagani D et al (2007) Bisphosphonate-associated osteonecrosis of the jaws: a therapeutic dilemma. Oral Surg Oral Med Oral Pathol Oral Radiol Endod 103(3):e1–e5
16. Neumann B, Gregersen H (2006) Bisphosphonates and osteonecrosis of the jaws in patients with myelomatosis. Ugeskr Laeger 168(21):2078–2079
17. Engroff SL, Coletti D (2008) Bisphosphonate related osteonecrosis of the palate: report of a case managed with free tissue transfer. Oral Surg Oral Med Oral Pathol Oral Radiol Endod 105:580–582
18. Stanton DC, Balasanian E (2009) Outcome of surgical management of bisphosphonate-related osteonecrosis of the jaws: review of 33 surgical cases. J Oral Maxillofac Surg 67:943–950
19. Nocini PF, Saia G, Bettini G, Ragazzo M, Blandamura S, Chiarini L, Bedogni A (2009) Vascularized fibula flap reconstruction of the mandible in bisphosphonate-related osteonecrosis. Eur J Surg Oncol 35:373–379

20. Bedogni A, Bettini G, Totola A, Saia G, Nocini PF (2010) Oral bisphosphonate-associated osteonecrosis of the jaw after implant surgery: a case report and literature review. J Oral Maxillofac Surg 68:1662–1666
21. Wongchuensoontorn C, Liebehenschel N, Wagner K et al (2009) Pathological fractures in patients caused by bisphosphonate-related osteonecrosis of the jaws: report of 3 cases. J Oral Maxillofac Surg 67:1311–1316
22. Vaszilkó M, Barabás J, Szabó G, Velich N, Cséplo K, Ujpál M (2007) Osteonecrosis of the jaws by using bisphosphonates. Fogorv Sz 100(3):115–119
23. Farrugia MC, Summerlin DJ, Krowiak E et al (2006) Osteonecrosis of the mandible or maxilla associated with the use of new generation bisphosphonates. Laryngoscope 116(1):115–120
24. Carlson ER, Basile JD (2009) The role of surgical resection in the management of bisphosphonate-related osteonecrosis of the jaws. J Oral Maxillofac Surg 67(Suppl 1):85–95
25. McLeod NM, Davies BJ, Brennan PA (2009) Management of patients at risk of bisphosphonate osteonecrosis in maxillofacial surgery units in the UK. Surgeon 7(1):18–23
26. Wutzl A, Biedermann E, Wanschitz F et al (2008) Treatment results of bisphosphonate-related osteonecrosis of the jaws. Head Neck 30(9):1224–1230
27. Marx RE (2009) Reconstruction of defects caused by bisphosphonate-induced osteonecrosis of the jaws. J Oral Maxillofac Surg 67(Suppl 1):107–119
28. Coletti D, Ord RA (2008) Treatment rationale for pathological fractures of the mandible: a series of 44 fractures. Int J Oral Maxillofac Surg 37:216
29. Adornato MC, Morcos I, Rozanski J (2007) The treatment of bisphosphonate-associated osteonecrosis of the jaws with bone resection and autologous platelet-derived growth factors. J Am Dent Assoc 138:971–977
30. Pirih FQ, Zablotsky M, Cordell K, McCauley LK (2009) Case report of implant placement in a patient with Paget's disease on bisphosphonate therapy. J Mich Dent Assoc 91(5):38–43

15 BRONJ: The Future

Salvatore L. Ruggiero

Abstract

Bisphosphonates are a class of agents that are widely used in the management of metastatic disease to the bone and in diseases of altered bone-turnover. Despite these benefits, bisphosphonate-related osteonecrosis of the jaw (BRONJ) has emerged as a complication that has afflicted a subset of patients receiving these drugs for the treatment of osteoporosis and metastatic bone cancer. The risk of developing this complication appears to be related to the potency of the bisphosphonate, the duration of exposure, and dentoalveolar trauma. Stage-specific management strategies have been developed as well as guidelines for evaluating the potential risks associated with this complication. In the past few years, based on the results of in vivo and in vitro research, there has been significant progress toward understanding osteonecrosis of the jaw. This chapter provides a review of the evolving strategies for the diagnosis, prevention, and management of BRONJ. New insights regarding the pathogenesis and treatment of this complication are discussed, as are the future challenges associated with the new drug regimens that have recently emerged for the treatment of osteoporosis and cancer.

S. L. Ruggiero (✉)
New York Center for Orthognathic and Maxillofacial Surgery,
Department of Oral and Maxillofacial Surgery,
Stony Brook School of Dental Medicine, Lake Success, NY, USA
e-mail: sruggie@optonline.net

F. S. De Ponte (ed.), *Bisphosphonates and Osteonecrosis of the Jaw: A Multidisciplinary Approach*, DOI: 10.1007/978-88-470-2083-2_15,

15.1 Introduction

Since the first description of bone necrosis in patients receiving bisphosphonate therapy, in 2003 [1], there have been multiple retrospective, prospective, and case-controlled studies that have served to characterize the diagnosis, associated risk factors, and treatment of this new complication known as bisphosphonate-related osteonecrosis of the jaws (BRONJ). This term was adopted by the American Association of Oral and Maxillofacial Surgeons in the original and updated guidelines paper, since it best reflects our current understanding of this process. This entity is also referred to as bisphosphonate-induced osteonecrosis of the jaw (BIONJ) and bisphosphonate-associated osteonecrosis of the jaw (BAONJ), which has created a level of confusion and inconsistency within the literature. However, in the very near future it is likely that all these terms will change in order to accommodate the new biological agents (denosumab), which have a similar potential to cause jaw necrosis but do not contain a bisphosphonate. While it was not the case 5 years ago, BRONJ is now a well-recognized entity that is associated with several risk factors that have been identified across various disciplines in medicine and dentistry. With this level of broad-based recognition, new clinical and basic-science research initiatives are likely to elucidate the etiopathogenesis of BRONJ and significantly improve disease management and prevention.

15.2 Basic Science and Research

Since BRONJ was first described [1, 2], the importance of developing an adequate animal model to study the factors associated with its etiology, presentation, and response to treatment has been realized [3, 4]. The challenge for any animal researcher is to establish a model in which the disease in the animal is analogous to the human condition in terms of bone healing and response to therapy. Such models also must take into consideration that bone remodeling in humans and large animal species occurs intracortically as opposed to at the bone surface.

In mouse models, bone-matrix necrosis and delayed extraction-socket healing have been demonstrated in animals exposed to zolendronic acid. Several studies have also focused on the rat model, in which exposed bone was noted in a large percentage of extraction sites in bisphosphonate-treated animals [5–7]. The results obtained with these models are certainly promising and may provide the groundwork for future experiments; however, a troubling issue for both rodent models is the fact that necrosis also developed in the control groups. Thus, the degree to which data from these animals can be applied to the biological system of a higher vertebrate remains to be established.

Osteonecrosis of the jaw (ONJ) has also been reported in a dog model in which animals that did not undergo surgery received various dosages of oral bisphosphonates over a three-year period. Although there were no areas of exposed bone, large regions of matrix necrosis were identified only within the alveolar bone of the treatment group [8]. Similar results were also obtained in dogs treated with an oral bisphosphonate for only one year [9]. In experiments specifically aimed at understanding the interaction between dental extraction and bisphosphonates in dogs, one out of six animals treated with intravenous zolendronic acid in doses and schedules comparable to those received by cancer patients developed exposed, necrotic bone at the extraction sites [10]. These findings in the dog model are encouraging and may lead to the development of a valid animal model for BRONJ. Equipped with an appropriate model, researchers will then be able to truly focus on the mechanism of BRONJ and establish the utility of preventive and management strategies.

15.3 Pathogenesis

Despite the fact that BRONJ has been well described in the literature, its pathogenesis remains poorly understood. Four major hypotheses have been proposed to explain the etiology of the disease: the suppression of bone remodeling (osteoclast-mediated), disturbances in bone vascularity (anti-angiogenesis), local mucosal toxicity, and genetic factors.

The most popular and researched of these hypotheses focuses on the profound inhibition of osteoclast function observed in BRONJ. Bisphosphonate-mediated suppression of bone remodeling is thought to have a more profound effect in the jaw, where baseline bone-turnover rates are typically 10–20 times greater than those of other skeletal sites. This position is supported by several studies that have demonstrated bone necrosis restricted to the alveolar component of the jaw in bisphosphonate-treated animals [8–10]. Recent reports of ONJ occurring in patients receiving anti-RANKL therapy have provided additional support for an osteoclast-mediated mechanism.

Defects in angiogenesis have also been considered as a mechanism underlying BRONJ. This has been fueled by reports of bisphosphonate-induced inhibition of angiogenesis in cell culture and in animal tumor models [11, 12]. However, these finding are tempered by other animal studies in which bisphosphonates had no effect on angiogenesis associated with endochondral ossification [13] and findings of normal vasculature in regions of bisphosphonate-induced matrix necrosis [8]. Direct mucosal toxicity from high bisphosphonate concentrations in the bone has been considered as the primary event for bone exposure and necrosis in the jaw [14]. This is based on cell culture data in which high concentration of bisphosphonates were found to be toxic to oral mucosal cells. In the clinical setting, such an affect would only occur if the oral mucosa were exposed to high concentrations of bisphosphonates for a prolonged period of time. This situation can theoretically occur at surgical sites or regions of inflammation, where there is a local reduction in the pH that in turn facilitates bisphosphonate release from bone [15]. However, the clinical scenario in which BRONJ presents spontaneously in the non-dentate region of the jaw is not consistent with this hypothesis.

The fact that only a small subset of patients exposed to bisphosphonates develops jaw necrosis has led some investigators to consider pharmacogenetic factors as well. Sarasquette et al. [16] noted certain genetic irregularities (i.e., single-nucleotide polymorphisms) in the cytochrome *P450-2C* gene in multiple myeloma patients with BRONJ. Those patients who were homozygous for the T allele had a 12.7 fold higher risk of developing the disease. The link to BRONJ formation includes alterations in bone vascularity and arachidonic acid metabolism, both of which are controlled by this gene.

All of these studies provide a much greater understanding of the BRONJ disease process and certainly point out the direction of future research. The degree to which any of these theories, working in concert or individually, can completely explain the development of this drug-mediated bone necrosis remains to be determined more fully. Considering the aforementioned studies, it is conceivable that a true and measureable level of risk may arise when factors such as jaw inflammation (trauma or infection), marker-gene expression, and anti-resorptive bone therapy are present.

15.4 Risk Factors and Clinical Diagnosis

The existing literature on BRONJ still does not support a causal relationship between bisphosphonate therapy and jaw necrosis. However, epidemiologic studies have established a strong association between intravenous bisphosphonates and BRONJ in the setting of malignant disease. This is based on a positive correlation between bisphosphonate potency and duration of therapy in relation to the presentation of BRONJ [17]. The same level of support does not exist for oral or intravenous bisphosphonates used in patients with osteoporosis or other non-malignant conditions. This is directly attributable to the fact that ONJ in the setting of oral bisphosphonate therapy remains a relatively uncommon event, and one that requires many years of drug-exposure. Therefore, prospective clinical studies aimed at determining accurate incidence/prevalence data or establishing valid risk factors will take many years to complete in addition to requiring a large number of study subjects. The cost and logistics of such a study will make its completion difficult.

The diagnostic criteria for BRONJ have remained unchanged since they were first defined in 2006. The tenants of the diagnosis include: (1) a history of bisphosphonates use, (2) exposed bone within the oral cavity, and (3) no history of prior radiation therapy to the jaws. However, the emergence of jaw necrosis in bisphosphonate-naïve patients receiving RANKL inhibitors [18–20] may necessitate a modification of these criteria. The finding of exposed, necrotic bone remains the hallmark of the diagnosis; therefore, the physical examination is the most effect method of establishing the diagnosis of jaw necrosis (Fig. 15.1).

A clinical staging system developed by Ruggiero [21] and adopted by the American Association of Oral and Maxillofacial Surgeons (AAOMS) in 2006 [22] has served to categorize patients with BRONJ, direct rational treatment guidelines, and collect data to assess the prognosis and treatment outcome in patients who have used either intravenous or oral bisphosphonates. Since the publication of these treatment guidelines, reports of non-specific signs and symptoms such as

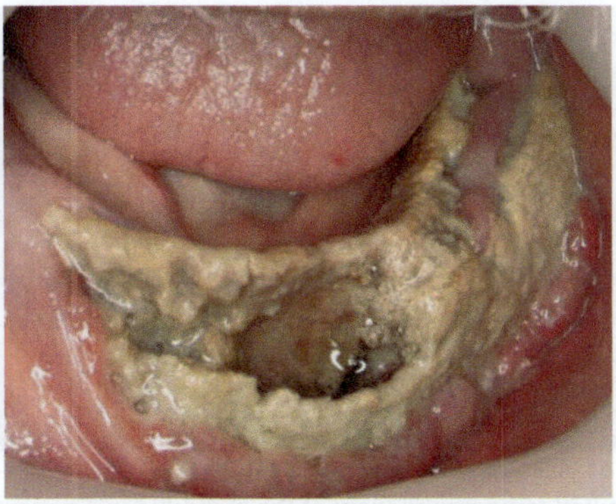

Fig. 15.1 Exposed, necrotic left mandible (BRONJ) in a patient with multiple myeloma and a history of zolendronic acid therapy

Table 15.1 BRONJ staging

At risk	No apparent exposed/necrotic bone in patients who have been treated with either oral or intravenous bisphosphonates
Stage 0	Non-specific clinical findings and symptoms such as jaw pain or osteosclerosis but no clinical evidence of exposed bone
Stage 1	Exposed/necrotic bone in patients who are asymptomatic and have no evidence of infection
Stage 2	Exposed/necrotic bone associated with infection as evidenced by pain and erythema in the region of the exposed bone with or without purulent drainage
Stage 3	Exposed/necrotic bone in patients with pain, infection, and one or more of the following: pathologic fracture, extra-oral fistula, or osteolysis extending to the inferior border or sinus floor

pain, abscess formation, altered sensory function, or osteosclerosis have emerged in patients with a history of bisphosphonate use but no clinical evidence of necrosis. In an effort to determine whether or not these findings represent a precursor for clinical disease, the recently updated AAOMS position paper has included these patients in a new stage 0 category (Table 15.1) [23]. The proportion of patients with stage 0 disease who will progress to overt BRONJ remains to be determined and represents an important area for future investigations.

Multiple risk factors, including drug-related issues (potency and duration of exposure), local risk factors (dentoalveolar surgery), local anatomy, concomitant oral and systemic disease, demographic factors, and genetic factors, have all been considered for this complication, but only three risk factors have remained constant throughout most clinical studies. In the majority of BRONJ cases reported to date, recent dentoalveolar trauma was the most prevalent and consistent risk factor [24–26]. Patients with a history of inflammatory dental disease, e.g., periodontal and dental abscesses, are at a seven fold higher risk for developing BRONJ [27].

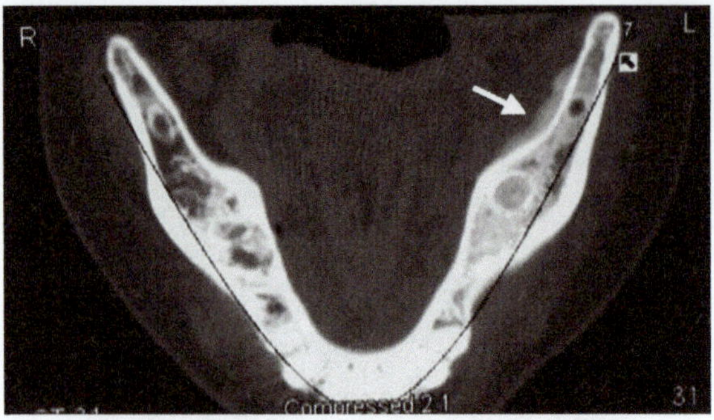

Fig. 15.2 Axial computed tomography view of the mandible in a patient with a history of breast cancer and established BRONJ. The *arrow* depicts an area of reactive periosteal bone formation on the lingual aspect of the left mandible

The duration of bisphosphonate therapy also appears strongly related to the likelihood of developing necrosis, with longer treatment regimens associated with a greater risk of disease development [26, 27]. In addition, the more potent intravenous bisphosphonates that are administered on a monthly schedule, such as zolendronic acid and pamidronate, are significantly more problematic than other preparations.

Efforts to establish risk assessment by measuring fluctuations in bone-turnover markers remain controversial [28–32]. The rationale for this approach is based on the knowledge that markers for bone remodeling will increase within months following withdrawal of oral bisphosphonate medications, suggesting a gradual normalization of osteoclastic function and bone remodeling [33, 34]. However, these markers are a reflection of total bone-turnover throughout the entire skeleton and are not specific to the maxilla or mandible, where it is suspected that the bone-turnover rate may be more severely depressed from prolonged bisphosphonate exposure. From a more practical perspective, using bone-turnover markers to estimate the level of bone-turnover suppression is only meaningful when the values are compared to baseline, pre-treatment levels, and these are rarely obtained in clinical practice. In addition, using the levels of bone-resorption markers to assess the BRONJ risk can be misleading in the small cohort of patients that develop osteoporosis despite normal baseline levels of these markers.

The radiographic features of BRONJ remain relatively non-specific. In fact, plain-film radiography does not typically demonstrate any abnormality in the early stages of the disease due to the limited degree of decalcification that is present. However, findings on plain-film imaging, such as localized or diffuse osteosclerosis or a thickening of the lamina dura (components of stage 0), may be predictors for future sites of exposed, necrotic bone. The findings on computed tomography (CT) are also non-specific but this modality is significantly more sensitive to changes in bone mineralization and therefore is more likely to demonstrate areas of focal sclerosis, thickened lamina dura, early sequestrum formation, and the presence of reactive periosteal bone (Fig. 15.2). CT images have also proved to be more accurate in delineating the extent of disease, which is very helpful for surgical treatment planning [35, 36]. The utility of nuclear bone scanning in patients at risk of BRONJ has received growing attention following reports of increased tracer uptake in regions of the jaws that subsequently developed necrosis [37, 38]. While nuclear imaging has limited value in patients with existing disease, it appears to have some level of potential benefit as a predictive tool in those patients with pre-clinical disease (stage 0) and therefore requires continued evaluation.

15.5 Treatment

The management of patients with BRONJ remains very challenging since surgical and medical interventions may not eradicate the disease. The goal of treatment for patients at risk of developing BRONJ or who have active disease is to preserve the quality of life by controlling pain, managing infection, and preventing the development of new areas of necrosis. This has to be balanced with the oncologic management of the patient with osteolytic metastases and with the risk of pathologic fracture in the osteoporotic patient.

The treatment approach for patients with stage 1 disease has remained primarily non-surgical since these patients do not have evidence of infection nor are they symptomatic. In most stage 1 patients, the exposed bone will eventually mature into a defined sequestrum that can be easily removed. Since infection and pain are typical for patients with stage 2 disease, these patients will benefit from local to systemic antibiotic therapy. They will likewise develop sequestrum, which in most cases can be managed with local debridement. In patients with stage 3 disease, the extensive nature of the necrosis and infection usually dictate early surgical treatment (segmental resection or marginal resection) for the control of infection and pain. Several institutions recently reported that early surgical treatment, regardless of disease stage, is associated with a good level of cure and disease control. This suggests that surgical treatment may soon play a larger role in managing this complication [39–41].

Alternative surgical and non-surgical approaches to treatment have recently emerged and may be of value. Hyperbaric oxygen therapy (HBO), as an adjunct to non-surgical or surgical treatment, is currently being evaluated at several institutions. The preliminary results from a pilot study suggest some improvement in wound healing and pain scores but the routine use of HBO as an effective adjunct or primary treatment modality requires further evidenced-based review [42, 43]. The use of platelet-rich plasma as an adjunct to local resection and primary closure was reported in a total of five cases at two separate institutions [44, 45]. In all instances, there was complete wound healing and resolution of pain. However, the small number of reported cases and the lack of controls mandate that further study of platelet-rich plasma is needed before it can be utilized therapeutically in BRONJ. In a single case report, the administration of systemic low-dose parathyroid hormone (PTH), an anabolic bone hormone, was successful in resolving an area of necrosis when other modalities of treatment had failed [46]. In a recent prospective, placebo-controlled study of 40 patients, low-dose systemic PTH in conjunction with vitamin D and oral calcium was associated with greater resolution of periodontal bone defects and accelerated intraoral osseous healing [47]. Although PTH is contraindicated in patients with osteolytic bone metastases, these promising findings may have real applicability for BRONJ patients in the non-cancer setting.

For those few patients who require surgical resection, the reconstruction of BRONJ-related defects has been challenging. Although there have been reports of immediate reconstruction with vacularized bone grafts, most surgeons are hesitant to proceed with such a procedure given the uncertain viability of the remaining native bone [39]. In those instances, the mandible is stabilized with a reconstruction plate and soft-tissue flaps [48]. The use of bone morphogenetic protein within a sponge carrier has been described for immediate reconstruction of discontinuity defects in BRONJ patients and might represent a viable alternative to conventional grafting techniques in this patient population [49].

If risk factors are truly predictors of disease, then modification of such factors should translate into a change (reduction) in disease severity or occurrence. In patients at risk of developing BRONJ, adherence to risk-reduction protocols has been reported to decrease the incidence of this complication [50]. Implementation of a detailed dental assessment and the avoidance of dentoalveolar surgery during treatment with zolendronic acid resulted in a five fold reduction of osteonecrosis [51]. In those instances in which BRONJ developed, the application of stage-specific treatment protocols resulted in a manageable level of disease and good symptom control in a large majority of patients [52]. Studies are underway at several institutions to determine whether dose-reduction schedules for zolendronic acid in the setting of cancer treatment will lower the incidence of BRONJ while retaining the oncologic effectiveness of the drug.

15.6 What We Don't Know

As we examine our present understanding of BRONJ as a therapy-associated complication and project our concerns into the future, there are many questions that remain to be answered. The recent emergence of anti-RANKL antibodies as a valid bone-targeted therapy for patients with cancer and osteoporosis has created a new set of potential challenges since these drugs also appear to be associated with the development of ONJ. While the reversible nature of this novel anti-resorptive therapy may prove to be uniquely beneficial in the management of affected patients, those potential benefits have yet to be studied or confirmed.

Accurate predictors of the disease also remain elusive. While certain types of nuclear imaging may prove to have some predictive value for those patients at risk, it is still not clear who should receive such a costly and invasive test or when it should be performed. As yearly zolendronic acid therapy (Reclast) becomes increasingly accepted, assessment of the risk of BRONJ takes on added urgency. Based on current studies, the risk of developing this condition was found to be very low through three years of bisphosphonate treatment [53, 54]. However, these data need to be compared with those from conventional oral bisphosphonate therapy in which a significant risk of developing necrosis only appears after a drug-exposure history longer than 3 years. More importantly, the risk of developing BRONJ in the setting of monthly intravenous zolendronic acid therapy for cancer has been well described. However, the degree and timing (if any) of risk-reduction following the cessation of therapy remain poorly understood. In addition, a better understanding of the exposure thresholds for intravenous (and oral) therapy is required so that patients and clinicians can be more accurately informed of the potential risks of these bone-targeted treatments.

First and foremost, our knowledge concerning the etiopathogenesis of this process, while much improved over the past several years, still has significant gaps. The identification of a reliable animal model system, based perhaps on one of the examples mentioned previously, will serve as a valuable experimental tool to assess theories of pathogenesis, analyze risk factors, determine the predictive value of diagnostic strategies, and evaluate treatment modalities. Since BRONJ has become a subject of great interest at national meetings and journal publications, awareness of this serious drug-related complication has certainly increased and will continue to do so throughout the dental and medical community. In updating dental and medical school curriculums, it will be important to include BRONJ at some point in training so that subsequent generations of health professionals are well informed and prepared to treat and care for these patients.

References

1. Marx R (2003) Pamidronate (Aredia) and zolendronate (Zometa) induced vascular necrosis of the jaws: a growing epidemic. J Oral Maxillofac Surg 61:1115–1117
2. Ruggiero S, Mehrotra B, Rosenberg T (2004) Osteonecrosis of the jaws associated with the use of bisphosphonates: a review of 63 cases. J Oral Maxillofac Surg 62:527–534
3. Bi Y, Gao Y, Ehirchiou D et al (2010) Bisphosphonates cause osteonecrosis of the jaw-like disease in mice. Am J Pathol 177:280–290
4. Kikuiri Y, Kim I, Yamaza T et al (2010) Cell-based immunotherapy with mesenchymal stem cells cures bisphosphonate-related osteonecrosis of the jaw-like disease in mice. J Bone Miner Res 25:1668–1679
5. Hokugo A, Christensen R, Chung EM et al (2010) Increased prevalence of bisphosphonate-related osteonecrosis of the jaw with vitamin D deficiency in rats. J Bone Miner Res 25:1337–1349
6. Lopez-Jornet P, Camacho-Alonso F, Molina-Miñano F et al (2010) An experimental study of bisphosphonate-induced jaw necrosis in Sprague-Dawley rats. J Oral Pathol Med 31:31
7. Maahs M, Azambuja A, Campos MM, Salum FG et al (2010) Association between bisphosphonates and jaw osteonecrosis: a study in Wistar rats. Head Neck 29:29
8. Allen M, Burr D (2008) Mandible matrix necrosis in beagle dogs following 3 years of daily oral bisphosphonate treatment. J Oral Maxillofac Surg 66:987–994
9. Burr D, Allen M (2009) Mandibular necrosis in beagle dogs treated with bisphosphonates. Orthod Craniofacial Res 12:221–228
10. Allen M, Kubek D, Burr D, Ruggiero S (2010) Compromised osseous healing of dental extraction sites in zolendronic acid-treated dogs. Osteoporos Int 22(2):693–702

11. Wood J, Bonjean K, Ruetz S (2002) Novel antiangiogenic effects of the bisphosphonate compound zolendronic acid. J Pharm Exper Ther 302:1055–1061
12. Fournier P, Boissier S, Filleur S, Guglielmi J et al (2002) Bisphosphonates inhibit angiogenesis in vitro and testosterone-stimulated vascular regrowth in the ventral prostate in castrated rats. Cancer Res 62:6538–6544
13. Deckers M, Van Beek E, Van Der Pluijm G et al (2002) Dissociation of angiogenesis and osteoclastogenesis during endochondral bone formation in neonatal mice. J Bone Miner Res 17:998
14. Landesberg R, Cozin M, Cremers S, Woo V et al (2008) Inhibition of oral mucosal cell wound healing by bisphosphonates. J Oral Maxillofac Surg 66:839–847
15. Otto S, Pautke C, Opelz C, Westphal I et al (2010) Osteonecrosis of the jaw: effect of BP type, local concentration, and acid milieu on the pathomechanism. J Oral Maxillofac Surg 68:2837–2845
16. Sarasquete M (2008) BRONJ is associated with polymorphisms of the cytochrome P450 CYP2C8 in multiple myeloma: a genome-wide single nucleotide analysis. Blood 111:2709
17. Dodson T (2009) Intravenous bisphosphonate therapy and bisphosphonate-related osteonecrosis of the jaws. J Oral Maxillofac Surg 67(Suppl 1):44–52
18. Stopeck A, Body J, Fujiwara Y (2009) Denosumab versus zolendronic acid for the treatment of breast cancer patients with bone metastases: results of a randomized phase 3 study. Eur J Cancer Suppl 7(2):2–3
19. Aghaloo T, Felsenfeld A, Tetradis S (2010) Osteonecrosis of the jaw in a patient on Denosumab. J Oral Maxillofac Surg 68:959–963
20. Taylor K, Middlefell L, Mizen K (2010) Osteonecrosis of the jaws induced by anti-RANK lingand therapy. Br J Oral Maxillofacial Surg 48:221–223
21. Ruggiero S, Fantasia J, Carlson E (2006) Bisphosphonate-related osteonecrosis of the jaw: background and guidelines for diagnosis, staging and management. Oral Surg Oral Med Oral Pathol Oral Radiol Endond 102:433–441
22. Surgeons AAOMS (2007) Position paper on bisphosphonate-related osteonecrosis of the jaw. J Oral Maxillofac Surg 3:369–376
23. Ruggiero S, Dodson TB, Assael LA et al (2009) American Association of Oral and Maxillofacial Surgeons position paper on bisphosphonate-related osteonecrosis of the jaws: 2009 update. J Oral Maxillofac Surg 67:2–12
24. Marx R, Sawatari Y, Fortin M (2005) Bisphosphonate-induced exposed bone (Osteonecrosis\osteopetrosis) of the jaws: Risk factors, recognition, prevention and treatment. J Oral Maxillofac Surg 63:1567–1575
25. Durie B, Katz M, Crowley J (2005) Osteonecrosis of the jaw and bisphosphonates (Letter). N Engl J Med 353:99
26. Badros A, Weikel D, Salama A (2006) Osteonecrosis of the jaw in multiple myeloma patients: clinical features and risk factors. J Clin Oncol 24:945–952
27. Hoff A, Toth B, Altundag K (2006) Osteonecrosis of the jaw in patients receiving intravenous bisphosphonate therapy. J Clin Oncol 24:8528
28. Bagan J, Jimenez Y, Gomez D, Sirera R (2008) Collagen telopeptide (serum CTX) and its relationship with size and number of lesions in osteonecrosis of the jaws in cancer patients on intravenous bisphosphonates. Oral Oncol 44:1088–1089
29. Kunchur R, Need A, Hughes T, Goss A (2009) Clinical investigation of C-terminal cross-linking telopeptide test in prevention and management of bisphosphonate -associated osteonecrosis of the jaws. J Oral Maxillofac Surg 67:1167–1173
30. Kwon Y, Kim D, Obe J, Yoo J (2009) Correlation between serum C-terminal cross-linking telopeptide of type 1 collagen and staging of oral bisphosphonate-related osteonecrosis of the jaws. J Oral Maxillofac Surg 67:2644–2648
31. Lehrer S et al (2008) Normal serum bone markers in bisphosphonate-induced osteonecrosis of the jaws. Oral Surg Oral Med Oral Path Oral Radiol Endod 106:389–391

32. Marx R, Cillo J, Ulloa J (2007) Oral bisphosphonate-induced osteonecrosis: Risk factors, prediction of risk using serum CTX testing, prevention, and treatment. J Oral Maxillofac Surg 65:2397–2410
33. Rosen H, Moses AC, Garber J et al (2000) Serum CTX: a new marker of bone resorption that shows treatment effect more often than other markers because of low coefficient of variability and large changes with bisphosphonate therapy. Calcif Tissue Int 66:100–103
34. Rosen H, Moses AC, Garber J, Ross DS et al (1998) Utility of biochemical markers of bone turnover in the follow-up of patients treated with bisphosphonates. Calcif Tissue Int 63:363–368
35. Treister N, Friedland B, Woo S (2010) Use of cone-beam computerized tomography for evaluation of bisphosphonate-associated osteonecrosis of the jaws. Oral Surg Oral Med Oral Path oral Radiol Endod 109:753–764
36. Arce K, Assael L, Weissman J, Markiewitz M (2009) Imaging findings in bisphosphonate-related osteonecrosis of the jaws. J Oral Maxillofac Surg 67(Suppl 1):75–84
37. Chiandussi S, Biasotto M, Cavalli F et al (2006) Clinical and diagnostic imaging of bisphosphonate-associated osteonecrosis of the jaws. Dentomaxillofacial Radiol 35:236–243
38. O'Ryan F, Khoury S, Liao W, Han M (2009) Intravenous bisphosphonate-related osteonecrosis of the jaw: bone scintigraphy as a n early indicator. J Oral Maxillofac Surg 67:1363–1372
39. Carlson E, Basile J (2009) The role of surgical resection in the management of bisphosphonate-relatred osteonecrosis of the jaws. J Oral Maxillofac Surg 67(Suppl 1):85–95
40. Mucke T, Koschinski J, Deppe H, Wagenpfeil S et al (2010) Outcome of treatment and parameters influencing recurrence in patients with bisphosphonate-related osteonecrosis of the jaws. J Cancer Res Oncol. doi:10.1007/s00432-010-0953-1
41. Stockman P, Vairaktaris E, Wehrhan F et al (2009) Osteotomy and primary wound closure in bisphosphonate-associated osteonecrosis of the jaw: a prospective clinical study with 12 months follow-up. Support Cancer Care 18:449–460
42. Frieberger J (2009) Utility of hyperbaric oxygen in treatment of bisphosphonate-related osteonecrosis of the jaws. J Oral Maxillofac Surg 67(Suppl 1):96–106
43. Sabino M (2007) Efficacy of hyperbaric oxygen therapy in bisphosphonate-related osteonecrosos of the jaw. J Oral Maxillofac Surg 65:S41
44. Curi M, Cossolin GS, Henrique Koga D et al (2007) Treatment of avascular necrosis of the mandible in cancer patients with a history of bisphosphonate therapy by combining bone resection and autologous platelet-rich plasma: report of 3 cases. J Oral Maxillofac Surg 65:349–355
45. Lee C, David T, Nishime M (2007) Use of platelet-rich plasma in the management of oral bisphosphonate-associated osteonecrosis of the jaw: a report of 2 cases. J Oral Implantology 32:371–382
46. Harper R, Fung E (2007) Resolution of bisphosphonate-associated osteonecrosis of the mandible: possible application for intermittent low -dose parathyroid hormone [rhPTH(1–340]. J Oral Maxillofac Surg 65:573–580
47. Bashutski J, Eber R, Kinney J, Benavides E et al (2010) Teriparitide and osseous regeneration in the oral cavity. N Engl J Med 363(25):2396–2405
48. Marx R (2009) Reconstruction of defects caused by bisphosphonate induced osteonecrosis of the jaws. J Oral Maxillofac Surg 67:107–119
49. Herford A, Boyne P (2008) Reconstruction of mandibular continuity defects with bone morphogenic protein-2 (rhBMP-2). J Oral Maxillofac Surg 66:616–624
50. Badros A, Evangelos T, Goloubeva O, Meiller T et al (2007) Long-term follow-up of multiple myeloma patients with osteonecrosis of the jaw. Blood 110(11):1030A–1031A
51. Dimopoulos M, Kastritis E, Bamia C, Melakopoulis I et al (2007) Decreased incidence of osteonecrosis of the jaw in patients with multiple myeloma treated with zoledronic acid after application of preventive measures. Blood 110(11):1056A
52. Mehrotra B, Fantasia J, Ruggiero S (2008) Outcomes of bisphosphonate related osteonecrosis of the jaw. Importance of staging and management guidelines. A large single institutional update. J Clin Oncol 26(Suppl):322

53. Grbic J et al (2010) The incidence of osteonecrosis of the jaw in patients receiving 5 mgs of zolendronic acid. Data from the health outcomes and reduced incidence with zolendronic acid once yearly clinical trials program. JADA 141:1365–1370
54. Grbic J, Landesberg R, Lin S (2008) Incidence of osteonecrosis of the jaw in women with postmenopausal osteoporosis in the health outcomes and reduced incidence with zolendroic acid once yearly. JADA 139:32–40

Index

F. S. De Ponte (ed.), *Bisphosphonates and Osteonecrosis of the Jaw: A Multidisciplinary Approach*, DOI: 10.1007/978-88-470-2083-2,

GPSR Compliance

The European Union's (EU) General Product Safety Regulation (GPSR) is a set of rules that requires consumer products to be safe and our obligations to ensure this.

If you have any concerns about our products, you can contact us on ProductSafety@springernature.com

In case Publisher is established outside the EU, the EU authorized representative is:

Springer Nature Customer Service Center GmbH
Europaplatz 3
69115 Heidelberg, Germany

Batch number: 10683214

Printed by Printforce, the Netherlands